THE

Science Backed

DASH DIET

MEAL PREP

FOR BEGINNERS

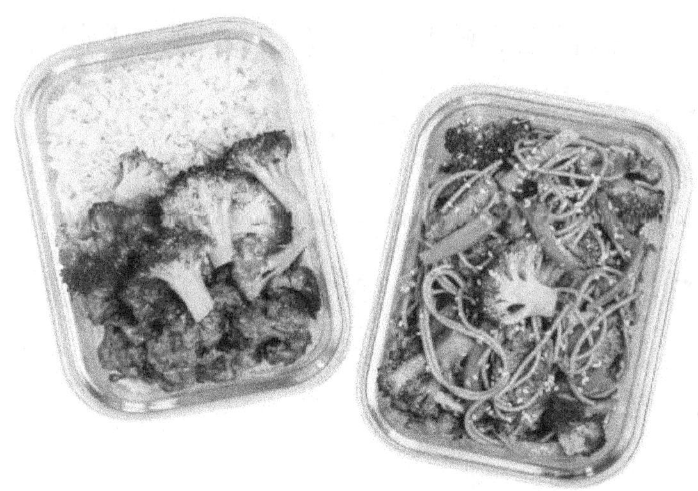

A Hassle-Free Guide and Simple meal plan to Prep ahead Recipes to Lower Your Blood Pressure & boost weight loss and improve your heart health.

Kelley Hamilton

Dedication

To all those who strive for a healthier tomorrow, May this book serve as a guiding light on your journey to wellness.

TABLE OF CONTENTS

Introduction

"Let food be thy medicine and medicine be thy food." Hippocrates once said something that has always struck a chord with me, particularly regarding health and well-being. I never expected my struggle and change to be the starting point of my DASH diet journey. I hope that this tale, together with the DASH diet's background and facts, will motivate and direct you toward improved health.

I was feeling scared and stressed while I was seated in a doctor's office a few years back. I had just received a diagnosis of hypertension, a silent killer of conditions I knew very nothing about. My physician discussed the dangers of uncontrolled hypertension, such as heart attacks, strokes, and renal damage. Those remarks had a profound impact on me and made me resolve to change.

When my doctor brought up the DASH diet, it was the tipping point. I had previously attempted several diets, many of which promised amazing outcomes but often left me feeling cheated and disheartened. But this time, things seemed to click. Dietary Approaches to Stop Hypertension, or DASH, was not your average diet craze. Prominent medical organizations such as the American Heart Association and the National Institutes of Health, supported it with strong research.

The National Institutes of Health financed several research that led to the development of the DASH diet in the early 1990s. The goal of the research was to develop a dietary strategy to counteract the increased prevalence of high blood pressure in the US. The Dietary Approaches to Stop Hypertension (DASH) trial, which showed that dietary modifications might considerably decrease blood pressure, was the result of their ground-breaking work.

A balanced and diverse intake of nutrients is the focus of the DASH diet, in contrast to many other restrictive diets. It is low in foods heavy in saturated fats, cholesterol, and salt and high in fruits, vegetables, whole grains, lean proteins, and low-fat dairy products. The first investigation yielded astonishing findings. In only a few weeks, those who followed the DASH diet had substantial drops in blood pressure that were on par with the effects of medication.

The DASH diet's common logic and simplicity impressed me as I learned more about its tenets. It was about constantly choosing healthy options rather than deprivation or extreme measures. I started to see food differently; instead of viewing it as an adversary to be avoided, I saw it as a potent ally on my path to improved health.

The DASH diet's emphasis on nutrient-rich meals that naturally decrease blood pressure is one of its most appealing features. Fruits and vegetables, for example, are rich in potassium, a mineral that helps regulate the body's salt levels and eases blood vessel pressure. While lean proteins and low-fat dairy products supply needed proteins and calcium without the extra fats that may contribute to hypertension, whole grains offer fiber and other key nutrients that support heart health.

As I began incorporating the DASH diet into my own life, I discovered that it included more than simply eating differently—it also required changing one's way of thinking. Rather than being a hassle, meal preparation turned into a thrilling task. I experimented with different recipes and ingredients, enjoying the deep, substantial flavor of lean meats, the satisfying crunch of healthy grains, and the vivid colors and tastes of fresh fruit.

My health suffered greatly as a result. My blood pressure started to decrease after a few months, and I felt more lively and invigorated than I had in a long time. Not because I was starving myself, but rather because I was giving my body the nourishment it needed, the weight I had been fighting to lose for so long began to slide away.

I also learned the value of moderation and balance from the DASH diet. It was about making better decisions and consuming a broad range of meals, not about eliminating whole food categories or strictly adhering to regulations. This method made it pleasurable and sustainable—a real lifestyle shift as opposed to a band-aid solution.

The flexibility of the DASH diet is what gives it its unique potency. The DASH diet's tenets are simple to implement into your everyday routine, regardless of your level of culinary experience. The recipes are simple and call for inexpensive, easily accessible ingredients. Your family will enjoy tasty, heart-healthy meals that you can prepare without having to be a gourmet chef.

A crucial element of the DASH diet is its focus on lowering salt consumption. Hypertension is mostly caused by high sodium levels, and processed and restaurant meals are heavy in salt in the average American diet. The DASH diet promotes the use of flavorings like herbs, spices, and other ingredients to improve food flavor without using salt. This offers up a world of culinary options and also lowers blood pressure.

I saw other good improvements in my life as I persisted in adhering to the DASH diet. I slept better, had more energy, and felt happier and more stable all around. I started to understand the link between nutrition and mental health, which supported the notion that our food choices had an impact on both our physical and mental health.

It wasn't always an easy path. There were moments when I battled cravings or had the need to go back to my bad habits. However, I remained motivated because of the information and comprehension I had acquired about the DASH diet. I discovered how to pay attention to my body's needs and recognize the food it requires to flourish.

Spreading the DASH diet to others was among the most satisfying parts of doing so. Inspired by my change, friends and relatives started enquiring and seeking counsel. I enjoyed seeing the wonderful effects of the DASH diet on their life and assisting them in learning about its advantages.

The DASH diet's effectiveness is proof of the value of evidence-based nutrition. It's about knowing the science behind what we consume and making wise decisions, not about gimmicks or fast remedies. Numerous people have seen significant changes in their blood pressure and general health, so the findings speak for themselves.

My aim in writing this cookbook is to impart the wisdom and experiences that have changed my life. To help you reach your health objectives and savor tasty, nourishing meals along the way, I want to provide you with the resources and direction you need to incorporate the DASH diet into your everyday routine.

This book's recipes are meant to be easy, approachable, and filling. They are a reflection of the fundamental ideas of the DASH diet, with an emphasis on complete, fresh meals that satisfy the senses and nourish the body. The DASH diet provides a sustainable and pleasurable route to well-being, regardless of your goals—whether you want to reduce blood pressure, shed pounds, or just feel better overall.

I want to encourage and enable you to take charge of your health, one meal at a time, via the pages of this cookbook. Although there may be difficulties along the way, the benefits will be incalculable. You may look forward to a brighter, happier future full of healthy meals and colorful tastes if you follow the DASH diet.

The Science Behind DASH: How It Lowers Blood Pressure

The Centers for Disease Control and Prevention state that "nearly half of adults in the United States suffer from hypertension." Although hypertension, or high blood pressure, is a significant risk factor for heart disease and stroke, there is good news: lifestyle modifications may control and even cure it. One of the best methods for lowering blood pressure and promoting heart health is the DASH diet, or Dietary Approaches to Stop Hypertension.

Early in the 1990s, scientists supported by the National Institutes of Health created the DASH diet. Their objective was to develop a meal regimen that would naturally lower blood pressure without the need for prescription drugs. The outcome was the DASH diet, which has been recommended by organizations and medical professionals worldwide ever since. The DASH diet's main tenets center on limiting meals high in added sugars, saturated fats, and salt and emphasizing foods high in minerals like potassium, calcium, and magnesium.

The DASH diet's focus on fruits and vegetables is one of its main components. Due to their high potassium content, these foods help reduce blood vessel wall tension and counteract the effects of salt. Several servings of fruits and vegetables each day are part of the DASH diet, which supplies potassium along with fiber, vitamins, and antioxidants that are essential for heart health. Bananas, oranges, spinach, and sweet potatoes, for instance, may greatly increase the amount of potassium you consume.

Another crucial element of the DASH diet is whole grains. Rich in fiber, foods such as quinoa, brown rice, oatmeal, and whole-wheat bread may lower cholesterol and lower the risk of heart disease. Important minerals, including iron, magnesium, and B vitamins, are also found in whole grains. Whole grains provide you with a sensation of fullness and satisfaction, which helps to control blood sugar levels and lessens the need to seek harmful foods.

In the DASH diet, lean proteins are also essential. Lean meats, poultry, fish, and plant-based proteins like beans, lentils, and nuts are all encouraged in the diet. Compared to red meats, these protein sources have less saturated fat and include vital amino acids that promote both general health and muscle repair. Because of its high content of omega-3 fatty acids, which have been shown to decrease inflammation and lessen the risk of heart disease, fish, in particular, is advised.

Dairy products with low-fat content are another crucial component of the DASH diet. These foods are great sources of calcium, which helps to control blood pressure, along with magnesium and potassium. You may be sure that you are getting adequate calcium without consuming the extra saturated fat that comes with full-fat dairy products by including low-fat or fat-free milk, yogurt, and cheese in your diet. For example, a serving of low-fat yogurt has probiotics, which support digestive health, in addition to calcium.

One important component of the DASH diet is cutting down on salt consumption. Elevated blood pressure and water retention might result from a high salt intake. The DASH diet suggests keeping daily salt consumption to less than 2,300 mg, with 1,500 mg being the best goal for those with hypertension. This may be accomplished by preparing meals at home using fresh ingredients, staying away from packaged and processed foods, and utilizing herbs and spices rather than salt to season foods.

Apart from these dietary recommendations, the DASH diet highlights the need for good fats. The diet promotes the intake of monounsaturated and polyunsaturated fats in place of saturated and trans fats, which are present in processed foods and red meat. Nuts, seeds, avocados, and olive oil are sources of good fats. These fats provide vital fatty acids that promote general health and assist in lowering harmful cholesterol levels.

The adaptability and inclusiveness of the DASH diet are among its advantages. Since it doesn't call for any particular meals or supplements, anybody may use it, and it's sustainable. The DASH diet encourages balanced meals and nutrient-rich foods, which decrease blood pressure while also improving general health. Rather than advocating drastic measures or short-term remedies, it supports mindful eating and long-term lifestyle adjustments.

Applying the DASH diet's tenets to everyday living may have a major positive impact on health. It provides a thorough nutritional strategy that lowers the risk of chronic illnesses, maintains heart health, and aids in weight management. Through comprehension and implementation of these concepts, people may proactively move toward improved well-being and a more promising future.

Benefits Beyond Blood Pressure: Weight Loss, Heart Health, and More

According to U.S. News & World Report, "the DASH diet is ranked consistently as one of the best diets overall." This praise is well-earned since there are other health advantages to the DASH diet (Dietary Approaches to Stop Hypertension) that go far beyond just decreasing blood pressure. Although the diet's main goal is to control hypertension, its all-encompassing nutritional approach also makes it an effective means of enhancing general health, facilitating weight reduction, and supporting heart health.

One of the main risk factors for cardiovascular illnesses, such as heart attacks and strokes, is high blood pressure, or hypertension. To counteract this silent killer, foods high in potassium, magnesium, and calcium were prioritized in the DASH diet, while those high in salt, added sugars, and saturated fats were restricted. As a consequence, one may have a longer and healthier life with a balanced diet that also helps decrease blood pressure.

The DASH diet's ability to promote weight reduction is one of its most notable advantages. The DASH diet promotes a balanced consumption of nutrient-dense foods, in contrast to many fad diets that emphasize severe calorie restriction or the elimination of whole food categories. This method naturally lowers cravings for unhealthy foods and increases fullness, which results in weight reduction. Because they are satiating and low in calories, fruits, vegetables, whole grains, and lean proteins make it simpler to maintain a calorie deficit without feeling deprived. This long-term approach to weight management helps avoid the "yo-yo" impact of dieting, in which people lose weight but quickly gain it back.

The DASH diet not only helps people lose weight but also greatly improves heart health. Dietary interventions that promote cardiovascular health also lower the risk of heart disease. For instance, whole grains provide a lot of fiber, which helps promote blood vessel health and decrease cholesterol. Antioxidants, which are abundant in fruits and vegetables, help shield the heart from inflammation and oxidative stress. Lean proteins, such as those from fish and poultry, further boost heart health by providing necessary amino acids without the additional saturated fat that comes with red meat.

The DASH diet's contribution to the prevention and management of diabetes is another important feature. The diet's focus on fruits, vegetables, and whole grains helps to enhance insulin sensitivity and control blood sugar levels. Compared to refined carbs, these meals have a lower glycemic index, which means that their effects on blood sugar levels are seen more gradually. For those who have type 2 diabetes or prediabetes, the

DASH diet is a great option since it may help control blood sugar levels and lower the risk of complications.

Another area where the DASH diet excels is in bone health. The diet has a lot of low-fat dairy products, which are high in calcium and vitamin D, two minerals that are necessary for strong bones to remain intact. A heavy fruit and vegetable diet also supplies potassium and magnesium, two elements that are essential for healthy bones. Together, these nutrients help preserve bone density and lower the incidence of osteoporosis, especially in the elderly.

The DASH diet has advantages for mental health as well. A diet high in fruits, vegetables, whole grains, and healthy fats may help elevate mood and enhance cognitive performance, according to recent studies. Antioxidants, fiber, and omega-3 fatty acids are among the elements in these meals that promote brain health and lower the risk of anxiety and depression. In addition, the balanced eating style of the DASH diet contributes to blood sugar stabilization, which may improve mood and energy levels all day.

Another area where the DASH diet is quite beneficial is in the area of digestive health. Constipation is warded off by the high fiber content found in fruits, vegetables, and whole grains, which encourage regular bowel motions. Additionally, fiber maintains a healthy gut flora, which is essential for immunological and general health. The DASH diet helps enhance food absorption and avoid digestive issues by supporting varied and balanced gut flora.

The DASH diet is notable for its accessibility and usefulness as well. Because it doesn't call for pricey supplements or unusual ingredients, it's a viable option for individuals of all income levels. The DASH diet is accessible to everyone, regardless of financial situation or culinary expertise, since it places a strong focus on whole, minimally processed foods. This pragmatism guarantees that everyone can benefit from the DASH diet, making it a genuinely inclusive and successful strategy for improved health.

In summary, the DASH diet has several advantages beyond only decreasing blood pressure, despite its well-known ability to do so. It aids weight reduction, heart health, diabetes control, bone health, emotional well-being, and digestive health by encouraging a balanced and nutrient-rich diet. One of the best dietary regimens out there is the DASH diet because of its realistic, sustainable principles and thorough approach to nutrition. Adopting the DASH diet may result in long-term advantages for the body and mind, including a life that is healthier, happier, and more energetic.

- How to Use This Cookbook

Chapter 1

Getting Started with DASH

Understanding the DASH Diet Guidelines

The World Health Organization states that "dietary choices can prevent more than 80% of heart disease, stroke, and type 2 diabetes." Dietary Approaches to Stop Hypertension, or DASH diet, is a shining illustration of how effective making the proper dietary decisions can be. The DASH diet was created to lower blood pressure, but it has now been shown to have several health advantages. Understanding the fundamental principles of the DASH diet, such as recommended foods, foods to restrict, and portion limits, is crucial to maximizing its benefits.

A range of nutrient-dense foods that support general health and reduce blood pressure serve as the cornerstone of the DASH diet. Paying attention to portion sizes is one of the main recommendations for ensuring a balanced diet without going overboard. Aim for six to eight servings of grains every day. One ounce of dry cereal, half a cup of cooked rice or pasta, or one slice of whole-wheat bread might all be considered single servings. Whole grains are best since they have more nutrients and fiber.

A staple of the DASH diet, four to five servings of vegetables should be consumed each day. This might be half a cup of cooked veggies or a cup of raw green vegetables. Vegetables are high in fiber, potassium, and magnesium—compounds that are essential for decreasing blood pressure. In the same way, four to five portions of fruits should be ingested each day. One medium fruit, a quarter cup of dried fruit, or half a cup of canned, frozen, or fresh fruit may all be considered serving sizes. These nutritious meals fulfill sweet cravings without sacrificing vitamins, minerals, or fiber.

Dairy products are necessary for their protein and calcium content, particularly if they are fat-free or low-fat. According to the DASH diet, one and a half ounces of cheese or one cup of milk or yogurt is two to three servings of dairy per day. It is advised to consume up to 6 ounces of lean meats, poultry, and fish per day, divided between two meals. This minimizes the consumption of saturated fat while ensuring an appropriate dose of protein. For example, three ounces of cooked beef, or about the size of a deck of cards, may constitute a serving.

Additionally stressed are legumes, nuts, and seeds, with four to five servings each week. A serving might consist of half a cup of cooked beans or peas, two teaspoons of seeds, or a third of a cup of nuts. These foods boost heart health and satiety because they are high in fiber, protein, and healthy fats. Good fats are important. Two to three servings of fats and oils per day, such as a tablespoon of oil or mayonnaise or a teaspoon of soft margarine, are advised. Monounsaturated and polyunsaturated fats from foods like avocados, almonds, and olive oil are the main emphasis.

Sweets and added sugars are permitted in moderation on the DASH diet, with a weekly maximum of five servings. This may be half a cup of sorbet or a spoonful of sugar, jam, or jelly. Here, moderation and selecting sweets with some nutritional value over empty calories are key points of focus.

The items to restrict are equally crucial. Less than 2,300 mg of sodium should be consumed daily; for those with hypertension, 1,500 mg is the optimal daily limit. This entails avoiding processed meals, which are often heavy in salt, and sticking to whole, natural foods. Cutting less on red meat and full-fat dairy products may help lower consumption of saturated fat. To reduce cholesterol and strengthen heart health, choose lean meats and low-fat dairy.

Reduce your intake of processed foods since they are usually heavy in harmful fats, added sugars, and salt. This covers products like fast food, snack foods, and soups in cans. Rather, cooking at home with fresh ingredients gives you more control over the components and guarantees that your cuisine meets DASH recommendations.

Moderation should also be applied to alcohol intake. It is advised that those who use alcohol limit their intake to one drink for women and two for men per day. Drinking too much alcohol may increase blood pressure and cause other health issues.

The DASH diet offers a well-rounded approach to nutrition when these rules are followed. It emphasizes nutrient-dense, low-harmful meals that support not just lowered blood pressure but also general wellness. Every food category is important for heart health, keeping a healthy weight, and supplying key vitamins and minerals. The DASH diet is a viable and sensible option for long-term health since it places an emphasis on portion management, which guarantees that nutritional demands are satisfied without going overboard. This nutritional strategy gives people the capacity to make educated decisions, which enhances well-being and lowers the risk of chronic illnesses.

Essential Kitchen Tools for Meal Prep

The ancient saying, ***"Failing to prepare is preparing to fail,"*** is particularly true in the kitchen. The correct equipment is needed for efficient meal prep to save time and guarantee consistent outcomes. These basic kitchen items may completely change the way you prepare meals.

An excellent knife set is essential. The majority of your chopping, slicing, and dicing tasks may be completed with a chef's knife, paring knife, and serrated knife. Accidents are less likely when cutting operations are done more quickly and safely using sharp blades.

A top-notch chopping board is an additional essential. For an adequate area for all your chopping requirements, choose a big, durable wood or plastic board. Keeping your cutting board clean also helps with cleanup and preserves your counters.

For precision, measuring spoons and cups is necessary. Accurate measurements guarantee that your recipes work out as written, particularly when combining or baking components. Purchase a dependable set that has both liquid and dry measurements in it.

It is essential to have a variety of sizes of mixing bowls. These are dishes for marinating meats, combining ingredients, and even serving. Bowls made of glass or stainless steel are enduring and simple to maintain.

Meal prep using a food processor may be revolutionary. You may save a significant amount of time by using it to quickly chop, slice, shred, and purée items. A food processor makes numerous activities easier, whether you're grinding nuts, cutting vegetables, or creating salsa.

To maintain the freshness of your prepared goods, storage containers are essential. Select airtight-sealed, microwave-safe, and BPA-free containers. Having clear containers makes it simpler to organize your cupboard and refrigerator since you can quickly see what's within.

And last, cooking may be made easier with a trustworthy slow cooker or Instant Pot. You can prepare meals ahead of time and have them ready when you need them thanks to this equipment. They are ideal for quickly preparing stews, soups, and other one-pot dishes.

Having these basic kitchen items can help you prepare meals more effectively and enjoyably, which will promote healthy eating practices and reduce stress while preparing meals.

Stocking Your Pantry: DASH Diet Staples

"A bank account is your diet. As Bethenny Frankel puts it, "Good food choices are good investments." This is especially true for those who follow the DASH diet. Keeping a well-stocked pantry guarantees that you can create nutritious, DASH-approved meals at any time. This comprehensive shopping list will help you stay on course.

The DASH diet's main component is whole grains. Keep supplies of whole-wheat pasta, brown rice, quinoa, and oats on hand. Due to their high fiber content and vital minerals, these grains help to maintain heart health and prolong feelings of fullness.

For plant-based protein and fiber, legumes and beans are essential. Have a variety of alternatives available, including kidney beans, chickpeas, lentils, and black beans. You may use them in salads, stews, soups, and side dishes.

Nuts and seeds are excellent as meal additions and snacks. Nuts like almonds, walnuts, chia seeds, and flaxseeds are great options. They may help reduce cravings for less healthful foods since they provide protein, healthy fats, and a delicious crunch.

Vegetables and tomatoes in low-sodium cans are handy for easy dinners. To limit your consumption of sodium, look for products without added sugar or salt. These may be used to give extra nutrients to casseroles, pasta meals, and soups.

Good oils to have in the cupboard are avocado and extra-virgin olive oils. The abundance of monounsaturated fats in these oils is good for the heart. Make marinades, and salad dressings, and cook with them.

Spices and herbs are key to flavoring food without raising the salt content of your diet. Garlic powder, onion powder, cumin, basil, oregano, thyme, and rosemary should all be kept on hand. These may keep your meals heart-healthy while also improving their flavor.

Stocks and broths low in salt are ideal for soups and stews. They enhance taste without having as much salt as many processed meals do. Choose broth that is lower in salt when it comes to vegetables, poultry, or meat.

Useful flours for baking and cooking include whole-wheat flour and other whole-grain flours like rye or spelled. Compared to their refined equivalents, these flours provide more fiber and nutrients, making them a better option for your favorite dishes.

Omega-3 fatty acids and protein are abundant in canned fish, including sardines, tuna, and salmon. Select kinds without additional salt that are packaged in water or olive oil. They go well with salads, sandwiches, or just by themselves for easy, fast dinners.

Having these DASH diet essentials in your pantry will ensure that you always have the supplies on hand to make a wide range of heart-healthy meals. In addition to meeting the

DASH recommendations, these basics make it simpler to eat a wholesome, delectable meal every day.

Tips for Successful Meal Prep

The famous words of Benjamin Franklin are "By failing to prepare, you are preparing to fail," and this is particularly true when it comes to eating a balanced diet. For anybody on the DASH diet, meal preparation may be a game-changer since it increases the likelihood of achieving dietary objectives by making wholesome meals more accessible. Here are some effective meal preparation techniques and their associated advantages.

Meal prep saves time, which is one of its main advantages. You may gain time during hectic workdays when making meals from scratch may not be feasible by setting aside a few hours each week for meal preparation. By doing this, you can make sure that you always have wholesome, DASH-friendly meals on hand, which will lessen the temptation to grab takeout or snack on convenience foods, which are sometimes heavy in fat and salt.

Plan your meals for the next week first. Make sure to include a range of fruits, vegetables, whole grains, lean meats, and low-fat dairy products in your breakfast, lunch, dinner, and snack choices. These foods are essential components of the DASH diet. Put your food plan in writing and make a thorough shopping list. A well-defined strategy guarantees that you purchase just what you need, cutting down on food waste and saving money. It also helps you keep organized.

Purchase high-quality storage bins. To accommodate various meal kinds and ingredient combinations, use a variety of sizes and shapes. Because they are odor-free, long-lasting, and microwave and oven-safe, glass containers are an excellent choice. To maintain freshness and prevent confusion, mark the meal and date on each container.

When preparing, concentrate on cooking in large quantities. Cook a tonne of grains (brown rice, quinoa, and whole-wheat pasta) and proteins (fish fillets, chicken breasts, and beans). You may also have flexible components for many dinners by roasting a large tray of mixed veggies. After cooking, portion these foods and keep them in your containers. In this manner, you may mix and match various ingredients to make well-balanced meals all week long.

To make your prepared meals last longer, use your freezer. Cooked grains, stews, casseroles, and soups all store nicely and reheat fast. Meals that are frozen in individual quantities make it simple to reach for a nutritious choice when you're pressed for time. Just be sure to properly mark everything with the contents and date to prevent mystery dinners.

Making parts that can be combined into various meals is another tactic. For instance, make a big pot of quinoa, roast a variety of veggies, and cook a batch of grilled chicken. You may mix and match these components to make your meals interesting and avoid monotony during the week. You may have quinoa salad with chicken and roasted veggies one day, and then use the same ingredients to create a filling wrap or soup the next.

Remember to bring snacks. Having wholesome snacks on hand is certain when you prepare them in advance. Chop up fruits and veggies, divide nuts and seeds, and prepare large quantities of nutritious dips, such as hummus or spreads made with yogurt. Keeping these snacks handy may prevent you from opting for less healthful foods when you're hungry.

A crucial component of the DASH diet is portion management, which is assisted by meal preparation. You may make sure you are consuming the appropriate quantities of each food category by pre-portioning your meals and snacks. This promotes weight control and helps you maintain a balanced diet.

Maintaining organization is essential. Stock your cupboard with DASH-friendly basics like healthy oils, low-sodium broths, canned beans, and whole grains. In this manner, you may effortlessly add more to your prepared meals as required. Keep your freezer and refrigerator organized as well, with distinct divisions labeled for various meal kinds and ingredients.

Because meal planning makes healthy eating more accessible and easy, it may greatly improve your adherence to the DASH diet. It guarantees that you always have wholesome meals available while also saving you time and lowering stress. Meal prep may develop into a beneficial habit that promotes your health and well-being with a little forethought and organization.

Chapter 2: Breakfast

As they say, "Breakfast is the most important meal of the day," and this is especially true for DASH dieters. A filling and healthy DASH breakfast provides vital nutrients and long-lasting energy, laying the groundwork for a healthy day. Lean proteins, like Greek yogurt or eggs, should be added after starting with nutritious grains like oatmeal or whole-wheat bread. Fruits and vegetables may also be added for extra vitamins and minerals. Maintaining good eating habits throughout the day is made simpler by balancing these components, which also helps to regulate blood sugar levels and reduce cravings in the middle of the morning. Accept the power of a balanced breakfast to get your DASH diet off to a great start.

**Smoothie Bowls**

Berry Bliss Smoothie Bowl

Prep Time: 5 minutes   **Cook Time:** none

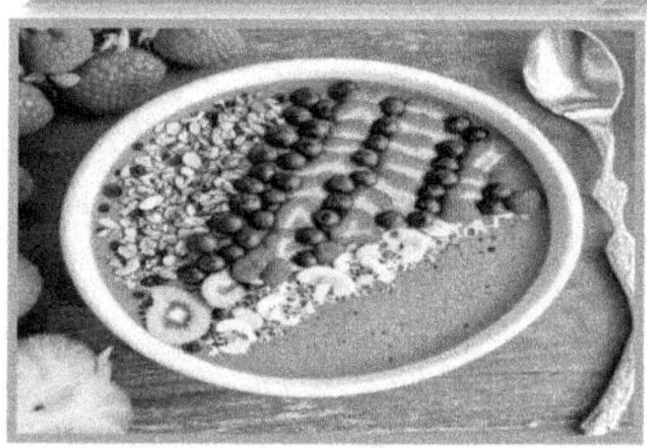

INGREDIENTS

- 1 cup frozen mixed berries
- 1 banana
- 1/2 cup Greek yogurt
- 1/2 cup almond milk
- 1 tablespoon chia seeds
- 1 tablespoon honey (optional)
- Toppings: sliced strawberries, blueberries, granola, coconut flakes

> Swap berries with tropical fruits like mango and pineapple.

INSTRUCTIONS

1. Combine the frozen berries, banana, Greek yogurt, almond milk, chia seeds, and honey in a blender.
2. Blend until smooth and thick.
3. Pour into a bowl and top with sliced strawberries, blueberries, granola, and coconut flakes.

Calories: 280, Protein: 10g, Carbs: 45g, Fat: 8g

Green Power Smoothie Bowl

Prep Time: 5 minutes   **Cook Time:** none

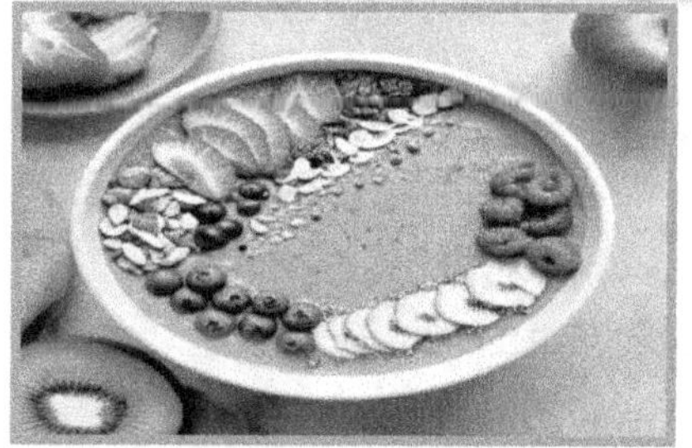

INGREDIENTS

- 1 cup spinach
- 1 banana
- 1/2 avocado
- 1/2 cup Greek yogurt
- 1/2 cup coconut water
- 1 tablespoon flax seeds
- Toppings: kiwi slices, chia seeds, almonds

> Use kale instead of spinach and add pineapple for sweetness.

INSTRUCTIONS

1. Blend spinach, banana, avocado, Greek yogurt, coconut water, and flax seeds until smooth.
2. Pour into a bowl and top with kiwi slices, chia seeds, and almonds.

Calories: 300, Protein: 11g, Carbs: 35g, Fat: 15g

Tropical Paradise Smoothie Bowl

Prep Time: 5 minutes   **Cook Time:** none hours

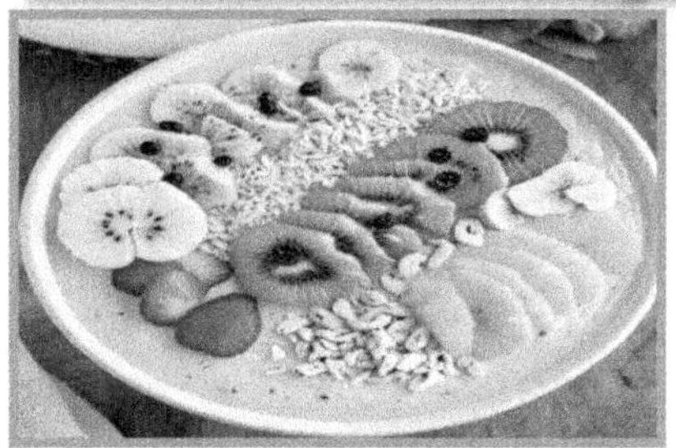

Add a handful of spinach for a nutritional boost.

INSTRUCTIONS

1. Blend mango, pineapple, banana, coconut milk, and Greek yogurt until smooth.
2. Pour into a bowl and top with shredded coconut, sliced banana, and chia seeds.

INGREDIENTS

- 1 cup frozen mango chunks
- 1/2 cup frozen pineapple chunks
- 1 banana
- 1/2 cup coconut milk
- 1/4 cup Greek yogurt
- Toppings: shredded coconut, sliced banana, chia seeds

Calories: 320, Protein: 8g, Carbs: 60g, Fat: 10g

Chocolate Peanut Butter Smoothie Bowl

Prep Time: 5 minutes   **Cook Time:** none

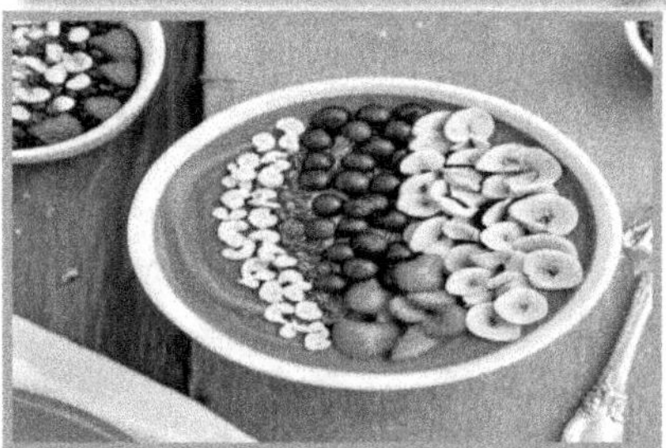

Use almond butter instead of peanut butter and add a handful of spinach.

INSTRUCTIONS

1. Blend banana, Greek yogurt, almond milk, peanut butter, and cocoa powder until smooth.
2. Pour into a bowl and top with sliced banana, granola, and dark chocolate shavings.

INGREDIENTS

- 1 frozen banana
- 1/2 cup Greek yogurt
- 1/2 cup almond milk
- 2 tablespoons peanut butter
- 1 tablespoon cocoa powder
- Toppings: sliced banana, granola, dark chocolate shavings

Calories: 350, Protein: 12g, Carbs: 40g, Fat: 15g

Acai Berry Smoothie Bowl

Prep Time: 5 minutes   **Cook Time:** none

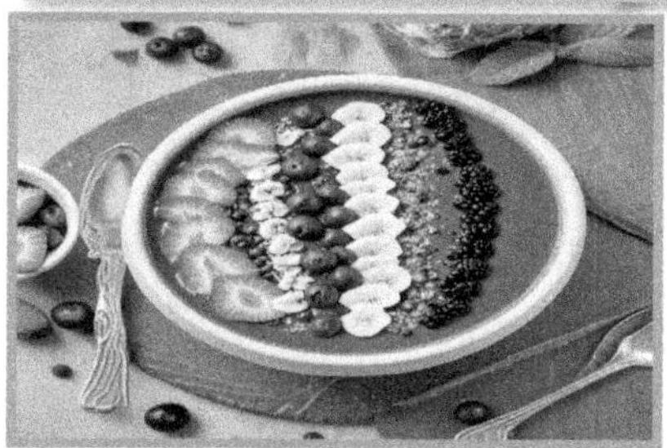

INGREDIENTS

- 1 packet frozen acai puree
- 1/2 cup frozen mixed berries
- 1 banana
- 1/2 cup almond milk
- 1 tablespoon honey (optional)
- Toppings: sliced strawberries, blueberries, granola, coconut flakes

INSTRUCTIONS

1. Blend acai puree, mixed berries, banana, almond milk, and honey until smooth.
2. Pour into a bowl and top with sliced strawberries, blueberries, granola, and coconut flakes.

Add a scoop of protein powder for an extra protein boost.

Calories: 290, Protein: 5g, Carbs: 55g, Fat: 8g

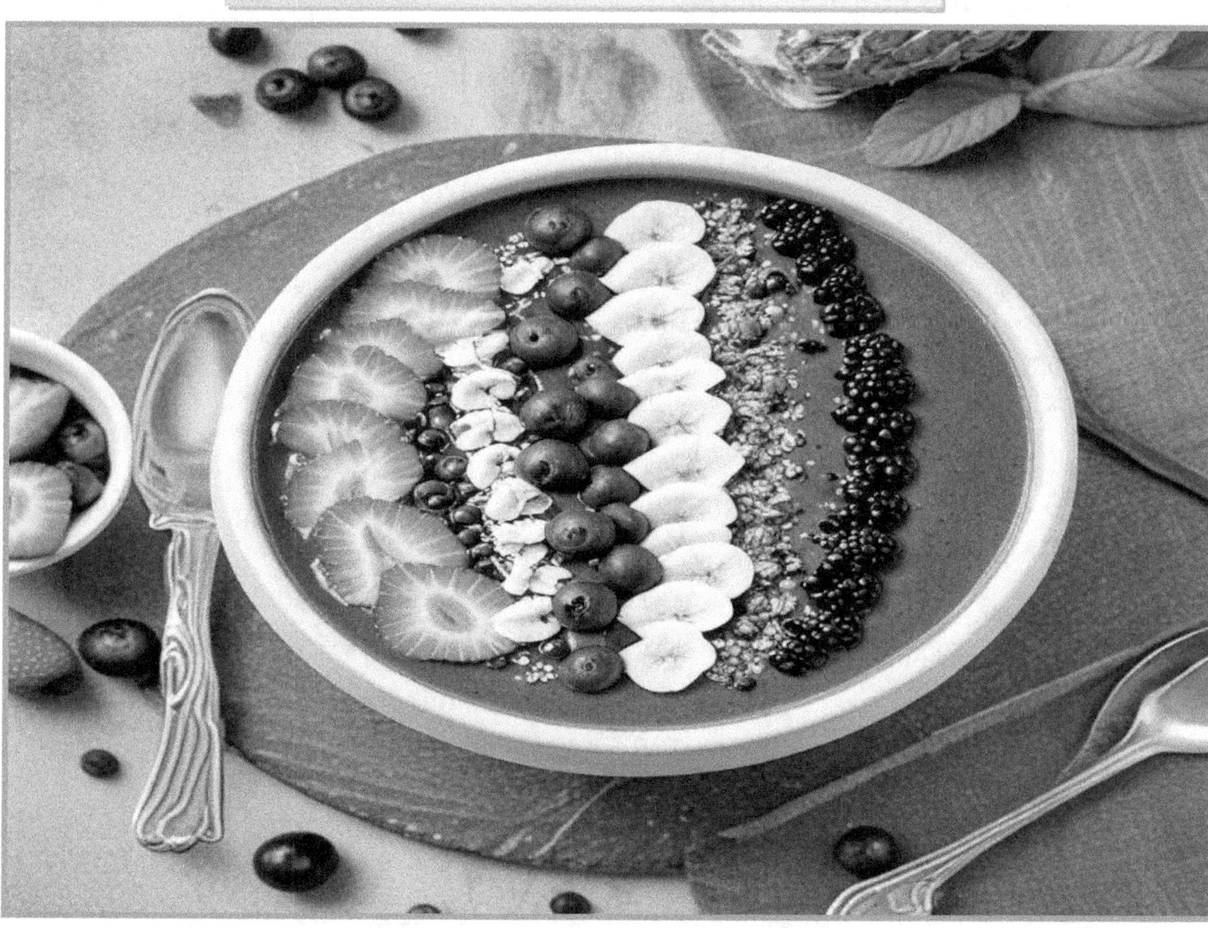

Classic Overnight Oats

Prep Time: 5 minutes   **Cook Time:** none

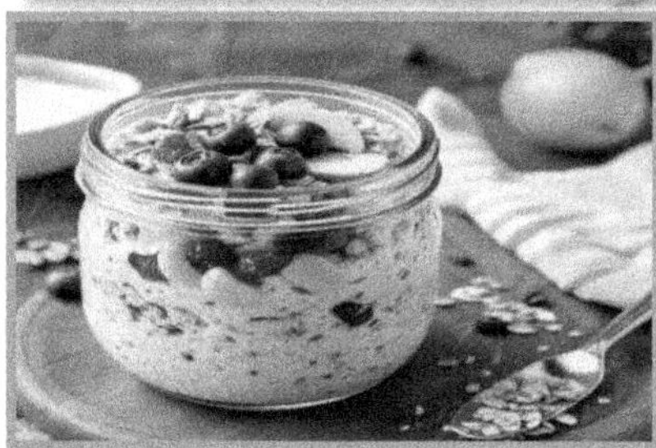

INGREDIENTS

- 1/2 cup rolled oats
- 1/2 cup almond milk
- 1/4 cup Greek yogurt
- 1 tablespoon chia seeds
- 1 tablespoon honey
- Toppings: fresh berries, nuts

INSTRUCTIONS

1. Combine oats, almond milk, Greek yogurt, chia seeds, and honey in a jar.
2. Stir well, cover, and refrigerate overnight.
3. Top with fresh berries and nuts in the morning.

Add a tablespoon of peanut butter or cocoa powder.

Calories: 250, Protein: 10g, Carbs: 40g, Fat: 7g

Apple Cinnamon Overnight Oats

Prep Time: 5 minutes   **Cook Time:** none

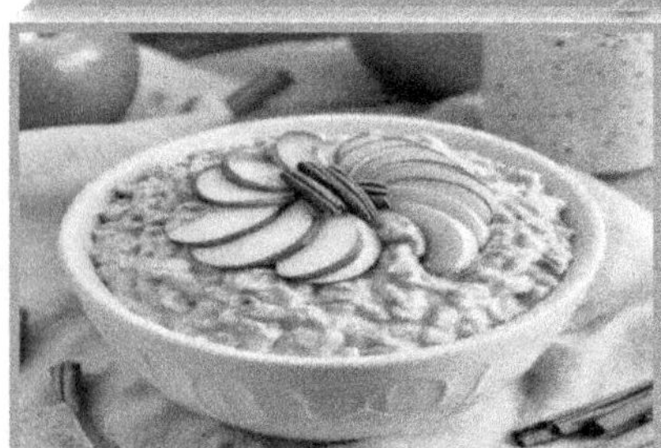

INGREDIENTS

- 1/2 cup rolled oats
- 1/2 cup almond milk
- 1/4 cup Greek yogurt
- 1/2 apple, diced
- 1/2 teaspoon cinnamon
- 1 tablespoon chia seeds
- Toppings: sliced almonds, extra apple pieces

INSTRUCTIONS

1. Mix oats, almond milk, Greek yogurt, diced apple, cinnamon, and chia seeds in a jar.
2. Stir well, cover, and refrigerate overnight.
3. Top with sliced almonds and extra apple pieces in the morning.

Add a tablespoon of maple syrup for extra sweetness.

Calories: 270, Protein: 9g, Carbs: 45g, Fat: 7g

Peanut Butter Banana Overnight Oats

Prep Time: 5 minutes | **Cook Time:** none

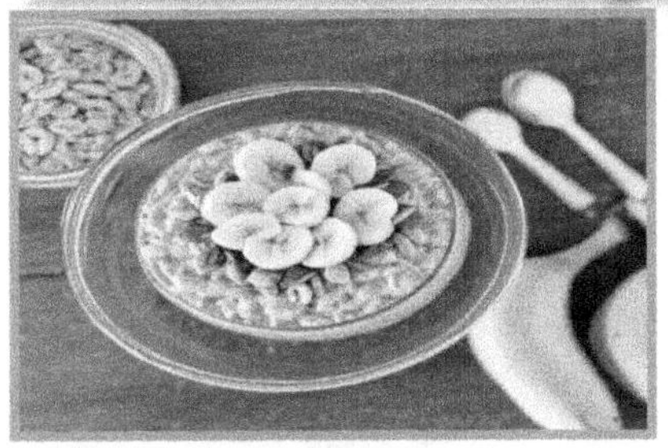

INGREDIENTS

- 1/2 cup rolled oats
- 1/2 cup almond milk
- 1/4 cup Greek yogurt
- 1 tablespoon peanut butter
- 1 banana, sliced
- 1 tablespoon chia seeds
- Toppings: extra banana slices, crushed peanuts

INSTRUCTIONS

1. Combine oats, almond milk, Greek yogurt, peanut butter, sliced banana, and chia seeds in a jar.
2. Stir well, cover, and refrigerate overnight.
3. Top with extra banana slices and crushed peanuts in the morning.

Use almond or cashew butter instead of peanut butter.

Calories: 320, Protein: 11g, Carbs: 50g, Fat: 10g

Chocolate Almond Overnight Oats

Prep Time: 5 minutes | **Cook Time:** none

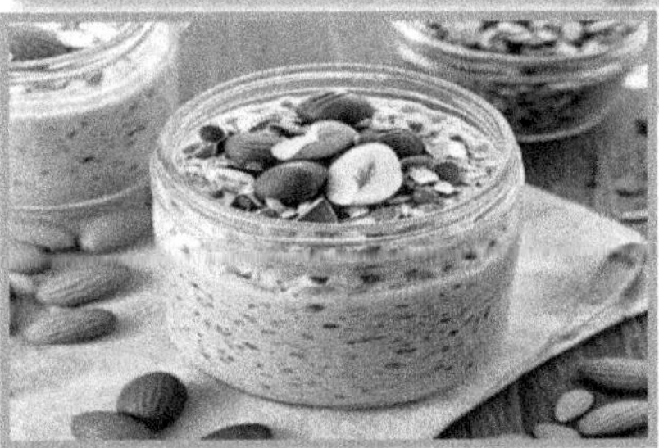

INGREDIENTS

- 1/2 cup rolled oats
- 1/2 cup almond milk
- 1/4 cup Greek yogurt
- 1 tablespoon almond butter
- 1 tablespoon cocoa powder
- 1 tablespoon chia seeds
- Toppings: sliced almonds, dark chocolate shavings

INSTRUCTIONS

1. Mix oats, almond milk, Greek yogurt, almond butter, cocoa powder, and chia seeds in a jar.
2. Stir well, cover, and refrigerate overnight.
3. Top with sliced almonds and dark chocolate shavings in the morning.

Add a teaspoon of vanilla extract for extra flavor.

Calories: 310, Protein: 10g, Carbs: 45g, Fat: 11g

Berry Vanilla Overnight Oats

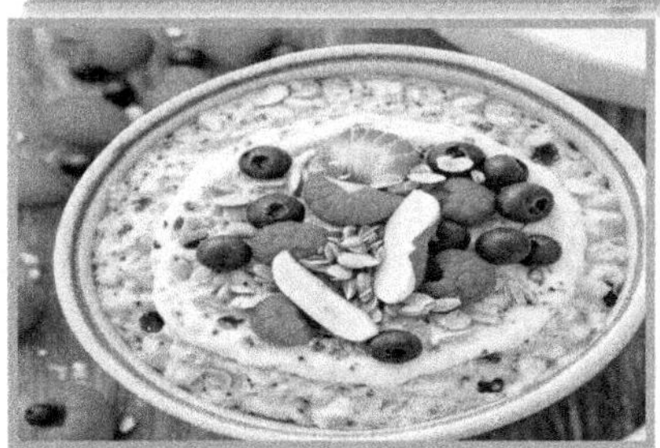

INGREDIENTS

- 1/2 cup rolled oats
- 1/2 cup almond milk
- 1/4 cup Greek yogurt
- 1/2 cup mixed berries
- 1 tablespoon chia seeds
- 1 teaspoon vanilla extract
- Toppings: fresh berries, granola

INSTRUCTIONS

1. Combine oats, almond milk, Greek yogurt, mixed berries, chia seeds, and vanilla extract in a jar.
2. Stir well, cover, and refrigerate overnight.
3. Top with fresh berries and granola in the morning.

Use different types of berries or add a tablespoon of honey for sweetness.

Calories: 260, Protein: 9g, Carbs: 45g, Fat: 6g

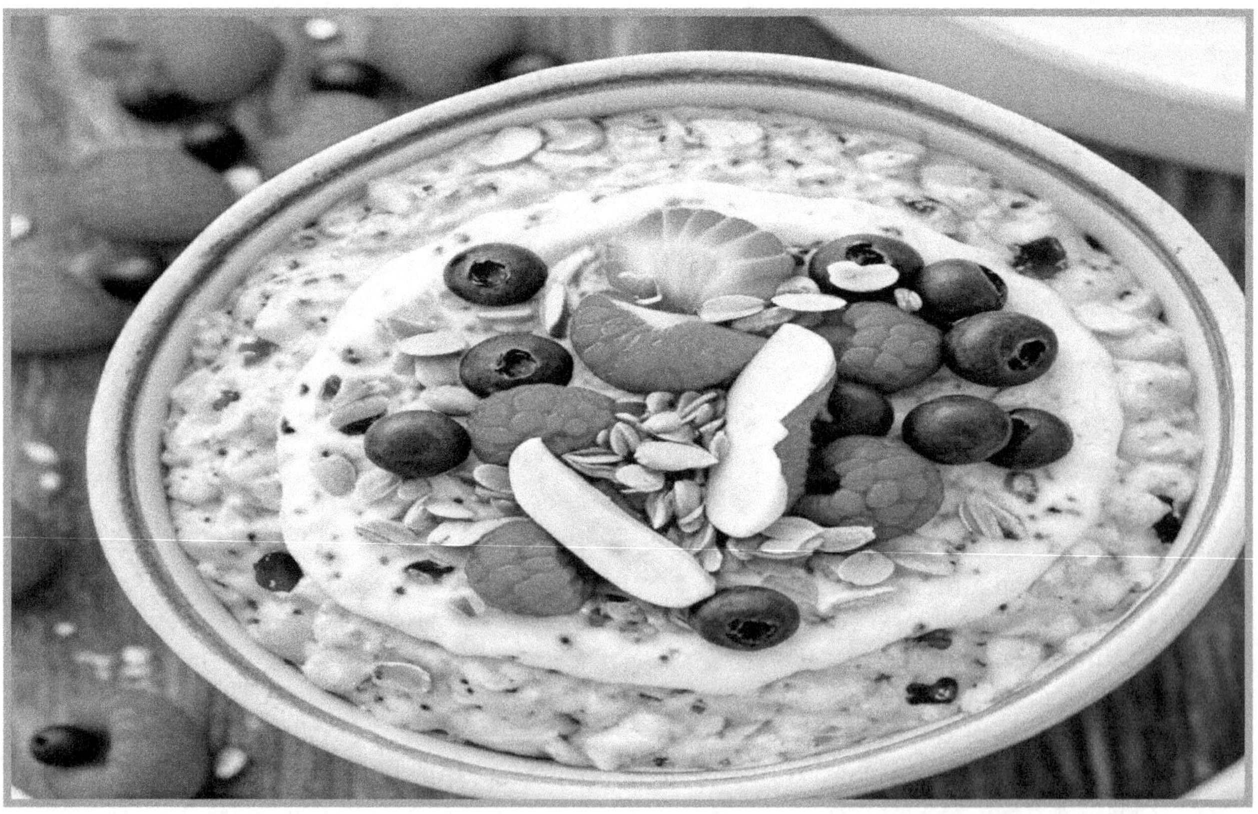

Blueberry Muffins

Prep Time: 10 minutes **Cook Time:** 20-25 hours

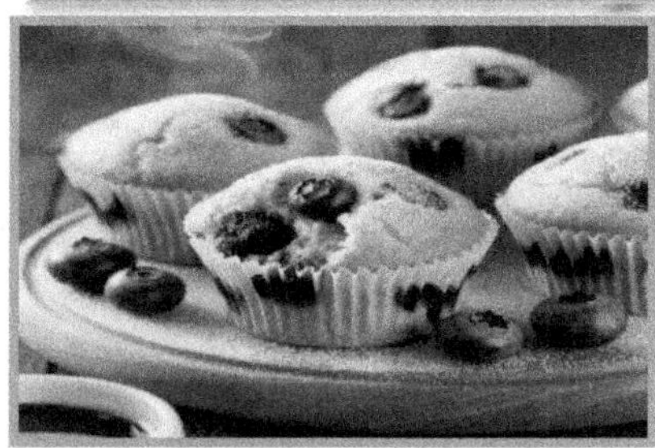

INGREDIENTS

- 1 1/2 cups whole wheat flour
- 1/2 cup rolled oats
- 1/2 cup honey
- 1 teaspoon baking powder
- 1/2 teaspoon baking soda
- 1/4 teaspoon salt
- 1 cup Greek yogurt
- 1/4 cup almond milk
- 1/4 cup coconut oil, melted
- 1 egg
- 1 teaspoon vanilla extract
- 1 cup blueberries

INSTRUCTIONS

1. Preheat oven to 375°F (190°C) and line a muffin tin with paper liners.
2. In a bowl, mix flour, oats, baking powder, baking soda, and salt.
3. In another bowl, whisk yogurt, almond milk, coconut oil, egg, and vanilla extract.
4. Combine wet and dry ingredients, then fold in blueberries.
5. Fill muffin cups and bake for 20-25 minutes.

Substitute blueberries with raspberries or diced apples.

Calories: 150, Protein: 4g, Carbs: 25g. Fat: 5g

Banana Bread

Prep Time: 10 minutes **Cook Time:** 55-60 minutes

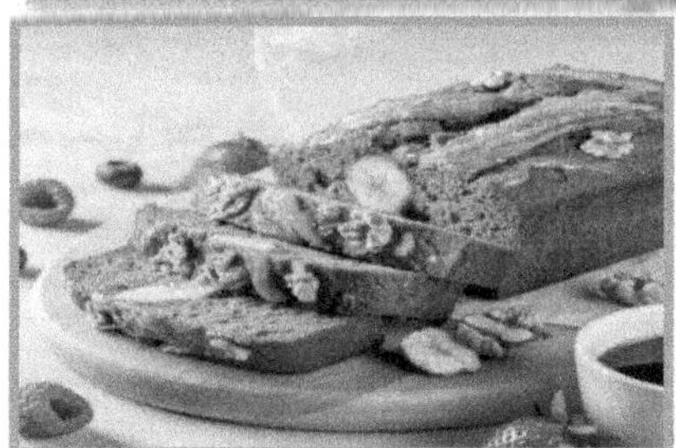

INGREDIENTS

- 3 ripe bananas, mashed
- 1/3 cup melted coconut oil
- 1/2 cup honey
- 2 eggs
- 1 teaspoon vanilla extract
- 1 3/4 cups whole wheat flour
- 1 teaspoon baking soda
- 1/2 teaspoon salt
- 1/2 teaspoon cinnamon

Add 1/2 cup chopped nuts or chocolate chips to the batter

INSTRUCTIONS

1. Preheat oven to 350°F (175°C) and grease a loaf pan.
2. In a bowl, mix mashed bananas, coconut oil, honey, eggs, and vanilla.
3. In another bowl, combine flour, baking soda, salt, and cinnamon.
4. Mix dry ingredients into wet until just combined.
5. Pour batter into loaf pan and bake for 55-60 minutes.

Calories: 180, Protein: 3g, Carbs: 30g, Fat: 6g

Apple Cinnamon Muffins

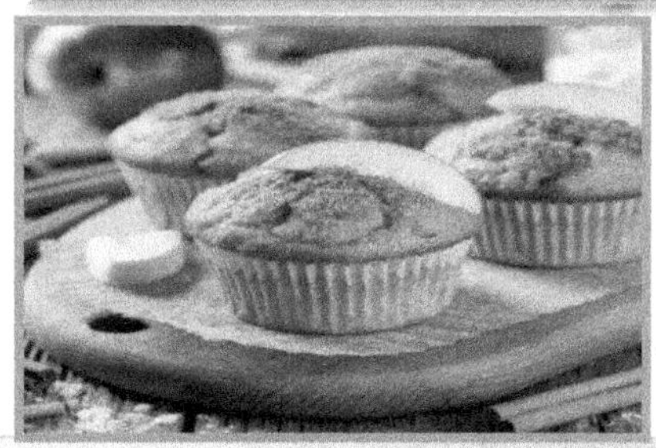

INGREDIENTS

- 1 1/2 cups whole wheat flour
- 1/2 cup rolled oats
- 1/2 cup honey
- 1 teaspoon baking powder
- 1/2 teaspoon baking soda
- 1/4 teaspoon salt
- 1 cup Greek yogurt
- 1/4 cup almond milk
- 1/4 cup coconut oil, melted
- 1 egg
- 1 teaspoon vanilla extract
- 1 apple, diced
- 1 teaspoon cinnamon

INSTRUCTIONS

1. Preheat oven to 375°F (190°C) and line a muffin tin with paper liners.
2. In a bowl, mix flour, oats, baking powder, baking soda, salt, and cinnamon.
3. In another bowl, whisk yogurt, almond milk, coconut oil, egg, and vanilla extract.
4. Combine wet and dry ingredients, then fold in diced apple.
5. Fill muffin cups and bake for 20-25 minutes.

Add a handful of raisins or nuts to the batter.

Calories: 160, Protein: 4g, Carbs: 28g, Fat: 5g

Carrot Cake Muffins

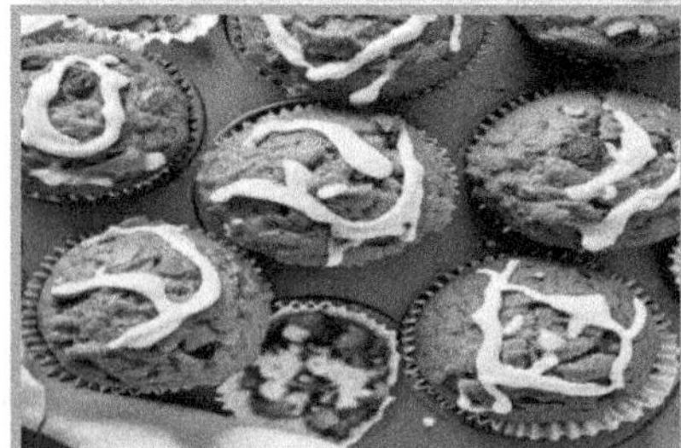

INGREDIENTS

- 1 1/2 cups whole wheat flour
- 1/2 cup rolled oats
- 1/2 cup honey
- 1 teaspoon baking powder
- 1/2 teaspoon baking soda
- 1/4 teaspoon salt
- 1 cup Greek yogurt
- 1/4 cup almond milk
- 1/4 cup coconut oil, melted
- 1 egg
- 1 teaspoon vanilla extract
- 1 cup grated carrots
- 1/2 teaspoon cinnamon

INSTRUCTIONS

1. Preheat oven to 375°F (190°C) and line a muffin tin with paper liners.
2. In a bowl, mix flour, oats, baking powder, baking soda, salt, and cinnamon.
3. In another bowl, whisk yogurt, almond milk, coconut oil, egg, and vanilla extract.
4. Combine wet and dry ingredients, then fold in grated carrots.
5. Fill muffin cups and bake for 20-25 minutes.

Calories: 170, Protein: 4g, Carbs: 30g, Fat: 5g

Zucchini Bread

Prep Time: 10 minutes   **Cook Time:** 50-55 minutes

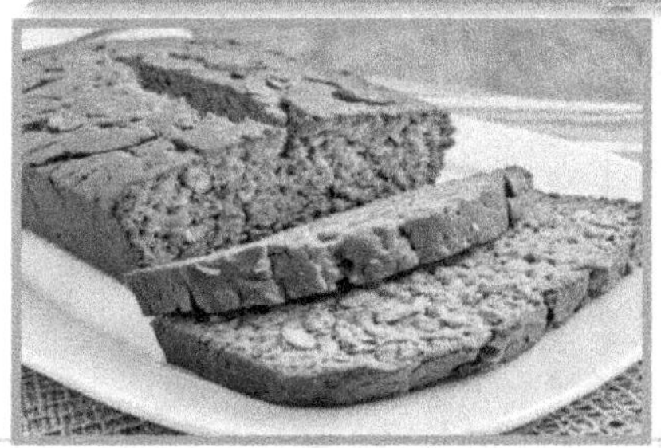

INGREDIENTS

- 1 1/2 cups grated zucchini
- 1/3 cup melted coconut oil
- 1/2 cup honey
- 2 eggs
- 1 teaspoon vanilla extract
- 1 3/4 cups whole wheat flour
- 1 teaspoon baking soda
- 1/2 teaspoon salt
- 1/2 teaspoon cinnamon

INSTRUCTIONS

1. Preheat oven to 350°F (175°C) and grease a loaf pan.
2. In a bowl, mix grated zucchini, coconut oil, honey, eggs, and vanilla.
3. In another bowl, combine flour, baking soda, salt, and cinnamon.
4. Mix dry ingredients into wet until just combined.
5. Pour batter into loaf pan and bake for 50-55 minutes.

Calories: 180, Protein: 3g, Carbs: 30g, Fat: 6g

Hearty Mornings

Veggie Omelet

Prep Time: 10 minutes   **Cook Time:** 10 minutes

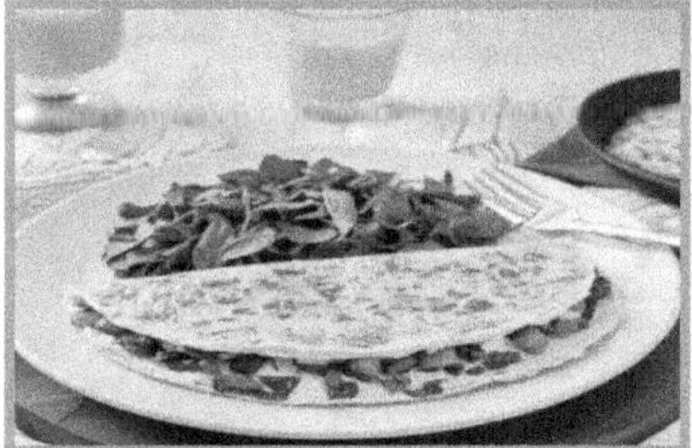

INGREDIENTS

- 3 eggs
- 1/4 cup milk
- 1/4 cup chopped bell peppers
- 1/4 cup chopped spinach
- 1/4 cup diced tomatoes
- 1/4 cup shredded cheese
- Salt and pepper to taste

INSTRUCTIONS

1. Beat eggs and milk in a bowl, then season with salt and pepper.
2. Heat a non-stick skillet over medium heat and add the egg mixture.
3. Add bell peppers, spinach, and tomatoes.
4. Cook until eggs are set, then sprinkle with cheese and fold.

Calories: 220, Protein: 18g, Carbs: 6g, Fat: 14g

Avocado Toast

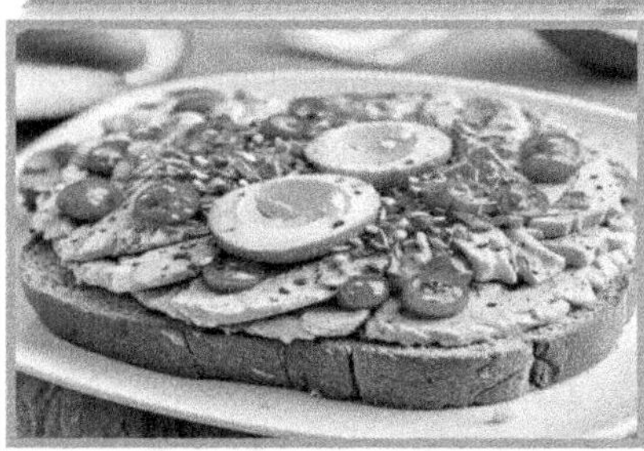

INGREDIENTS

- 1 slice whole-grain bread
- 1/2 avocado, mashed
- 1 egg, poached
- Salt, pepper, and red pepper flakes to taste

INSTRUCTIONS

1. Toast the bread slice.
2. Spread mashed avocado on the toast.
3. Top with poached egg and season with salt, pepper, and red pepper flakes.

Calories: 250, Protein: 10g, Carbs: 20g, Fat: 15g

Greek Yogurt Parfait

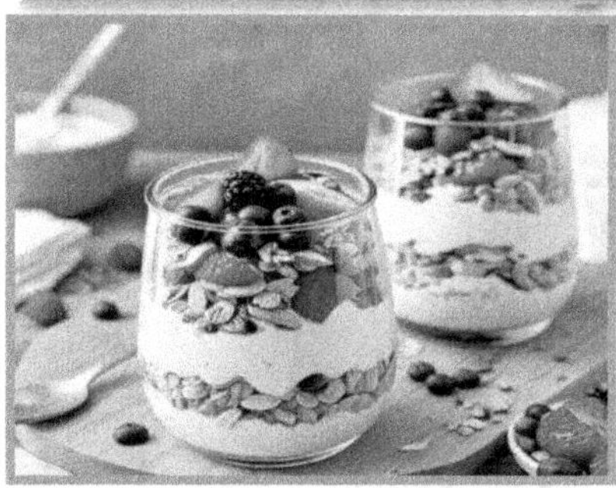

INGREDIENTS

- 1 cup Greek yogurt
- 1/2 cup mixed berries
- 1/4 cup granola
- 1 tablespoon honey

INSTRUCTIONS

1. Layer Greek yogurt, berries, and granola in a bowl.
2. Drizzle with honey.

Calories: 300, Protein: 15g, Carbs: 45g, Fat: 7g

Breakfast Burrito

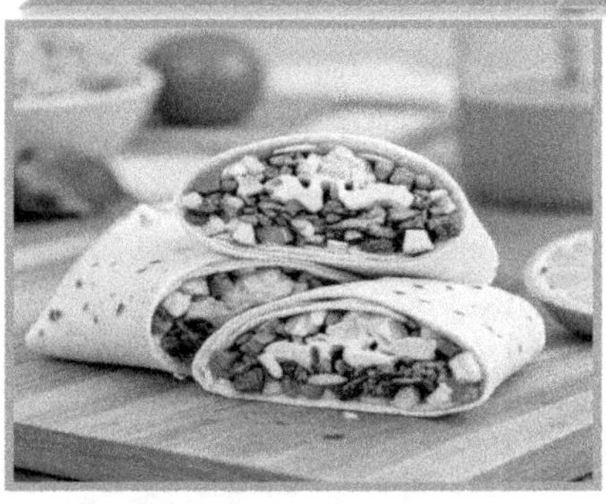

INSTRUCTIONS

1. Fill tortilla with scrambled eggs, black beans, tomatoes, and cheese.
2. Roll up and top with salsa and avocado slices.

INGREDIENTS

- 1 whole-wheat tortilla
- 2 scrambled eggs
- 1/4 cup black beans
- 1/4 cup diced tomatoes
- 1/4 cup shredded cheese
- Salsa and avocado slices for topping

Calories: 350, Protein: 20g, Carbs: 40g, Fat: 15g

Steel-Cut Oats

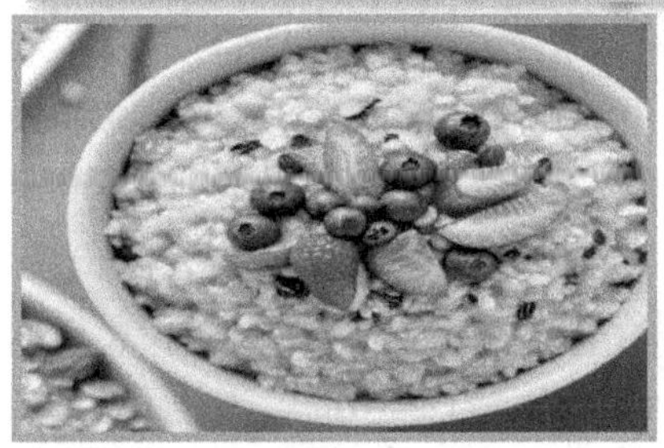

INSTRUCTIONS

1. Combine oats, water, milk, and salt in a pot and bring to a boil.
2. Reduce heat and simmer for 20-25 minutes, stirring occasionally.
3. Top with fresh berries, nuts, and honey.

INGREDIENTS

- 1 cup steel-cut oats
- 3 cups water
- 1/4 cup milk
- 1/4 teaspoon salt
- Toppings: fresh berries, nuts, honey

Calories: 250, Protein: 6g, Carbs: 50g, Fat: 5g

Chapter 3: Lunch

Many dietitians assert that "eating a nutritious lunch is key to sustaining energy and focus throughout the day." Vegetables, lean meats, and healthy grains are expertly balanced in a DASH diet meal to keep you feeling full and content while supporting weight control and heart health. The main goal is to include a range of veggies as they are a good source of fiber, vitamins, and minerals. Choosing nutrient-dense veggies such as broccoli, bell peppers, and leafy greens will give your meal more substance without adding too many calories.

For a DASH diet lunch, lean proteins such as grilled chicken, tofu, or lentils are essential. These proteins prevent hunger in addition to aiding in muscle development and repair. Choosing plant-based proteins such as chickpeas and lentils may also help decrease cholesterol, which is in line with the objectives of the DASH diet.

Another essential component of a healthy DASH diet meal is whole grains. Rich in fiber and complex carbs, foods like quinoa, brown rice, and whole-wheat pasta provide sustained energy and facilitate better digestion. By stabilizing blood sugar levels, these grains help avoid energy dumps in the middle of the day.

When these components are combined, a DASH diet lunch promotes general health while providing you with a satisfying and nourishing meal. It is simpler to follow this heart-healthy eating plan when there is a broad range of colors and textures in the meal. This also guarantees a wide range of nutrients.

Fresh Salads

Greek Salad

Prep Time: 10 minutes **Cook Time:** none

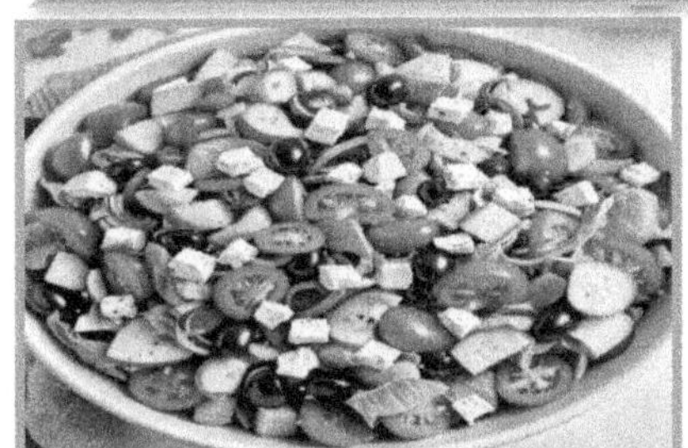

INGREDIENTS

- 1 cup cherry tomatoes, halved
- 1 cucumber, diced
- 1/4 cup red onion, thinly sliced
- 1/2 cup Kalamata olives
- 1/4 cup feta cheese, crumbled
- 2 tbsp olive oil
- 1 tbsp red wine vinegar
- 1 tsp dried oregano
- Salt and pepper to taste

INSTRUCTIONS

1. Combine tomatoes, cucumber, red onion, olives, and feta cheese in a bowl.
2. In a small bowl, whisk together olive oil, vinegar, oregano, salt, and pepper.
3. Drizzle dressing over the salad and toss to coat.

Calories: 200, Protein: 5g, Carbs: 10g, Fat: 15g

Spinach and Strawberry Salad

Prep Time: 10 minutes **Cook Time:** 10 minutes

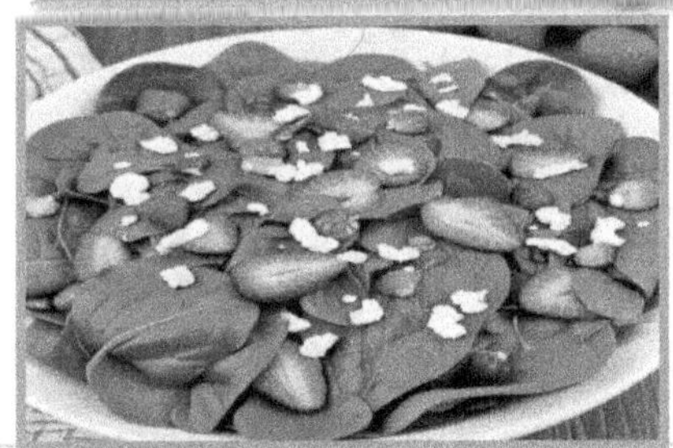

INGREDIENTS

- 4 cups baby spinach
- 1 cup sliced strawberries
- 1/4 cup sliced almonds
- 1/4 cup crumbled goat cheese
- 2 tbsp balsamic vinaigrette

INSTRUCTIONS

1. Toss spinach, strawberries, almonds, and goat cheese in a large bowl.
2. Drizzle with balsamic vinaigrette and toss gently to combine.

Calories: 180, Protein: 5g, Carbs: 15g, Fat: 12g

Chicken Caesar Salad

Prep Time: 10 minutes   **Cook Time:** 10 minutes

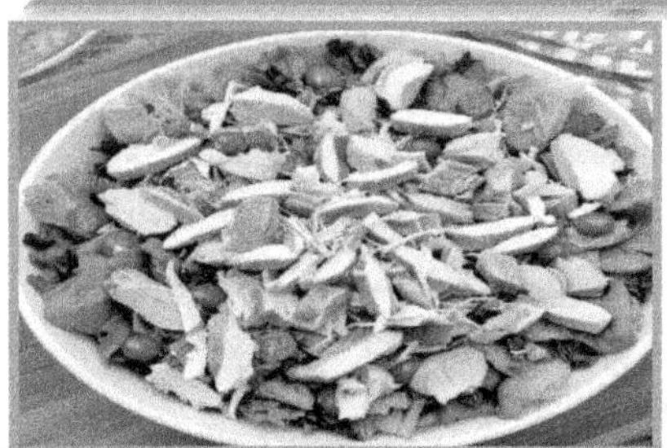

INSTRUCTIONS

1. In a bowl, combine lettuce, chicken, Parmesan, and croutons.
2. Drizzle with Caesar dressing and toss to coat.

INGREDIENTS

- 2 cups romaine lettuce, chopped
- 1 grilled chicken breast, sliced
- 1/4 cup grated Parmesan cheese
- 1/2 cup croutons
- 2 tbsp Caesar dressing

Calories: 350, Protein: 30g, Carbs: 20g, Fat: 15g

Quinoa and Black Bean Salad

Prep Time: 10 minutes   **Cook Time:** 15 minutes

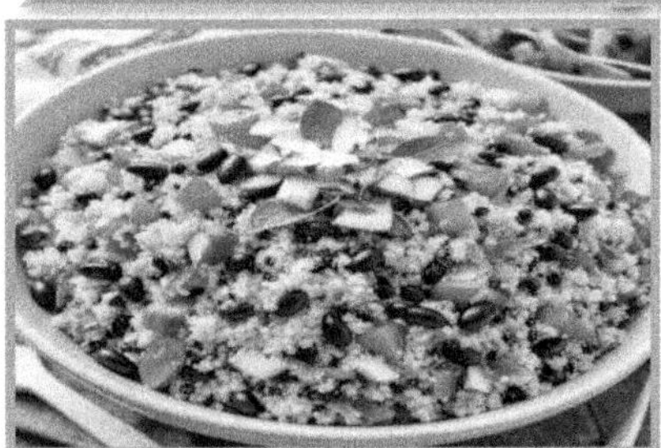

INSTRUCTIONS

1. Combine quinoa, black beans, corn, bell pepper, and cilantro in a bowl.
2. Whisk lime juice, olive oil, salt, and pepper in a small bowl.
3. Pour dressing over salad and toss to coat.

INGREDIENTS

- 1 cup cooked quinoa
- 1/2 cup black beans, rinsed and drained
- 1/2 cup corn kernels
- 1/4 cup diced red bell pepper
- 1/4 cup chopped cilantro
- 2 tbsp lime juice
- 1 tbsp olive oil
- Salt and pepper to taste

Calories: 220, Protein: 7g, Carbs: 30g, Fat: 8g

Caprese Salad

Prep Time: 10 minutes   **Cook Time:** none

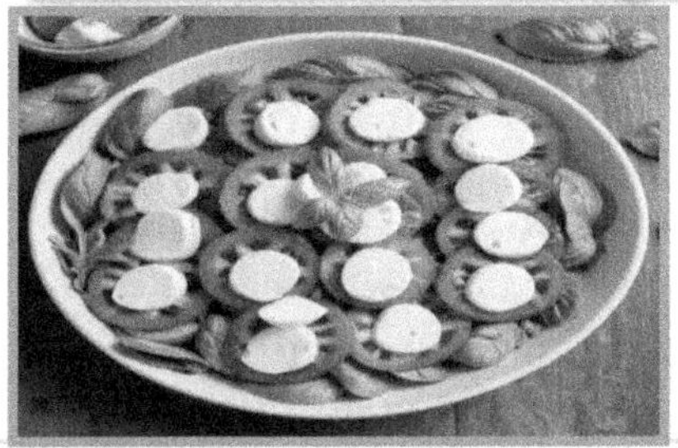

INSTRUCTIONS

1. Combine tomatoes, mozzarella, and basil in a bowl.
2. Drizzle with olive oil and balsamic vinegar.
3. Season with salt and pepper and toss gently.

INGREDIENTS

- 2 cups cherry tomatoes, halved
- 1 cup mozzarella balls
- 1/4 cup fresh basil leaves
- 2 tbsp olive oil
- 1 tbsp balsamic vinegar
- Salt and pepper to taste

Calories: 250, Protein: 12g, Carbs: 10g, Fat: 18g

Hearty Soups

Lentil Soup

Prep Time: 10 minutes   **Cook Time:** 30 minutes

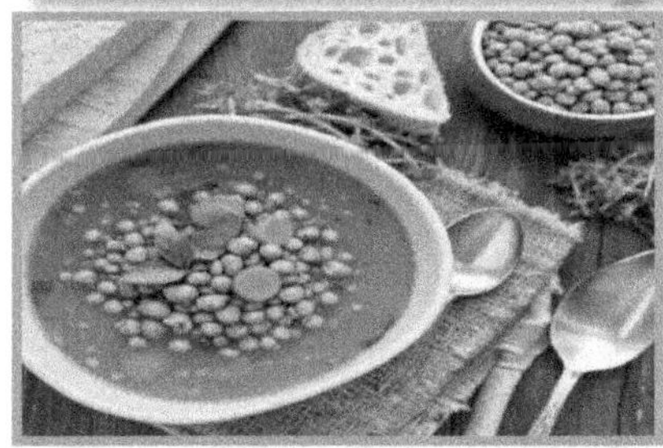

INSTRUCTIONS

1. In a pot, sauté onion, carrots, and celery until softened.
2. Add garlic and cook for another minute.
3. Add lentils, tomatoes, broth, cumin, salt, and pepper.
4. Bring to a boil, then simmer for 30 minutes.

INGREDIENTS

- 1 cup lentils, rinsed
- 1 onion, diced
- 2 carrots, diced
- 2 celery stalks, diced
- 3 garlic cloves, minced
- 1 can diced tomatoes
- 4 cups vegetable broth
- 1 tsp cumin
- Salt and pepper to taste

    Calories: 250, Protein: 15g, Carbs: 40g, Fat: 3g

Chicken Noodle Soup

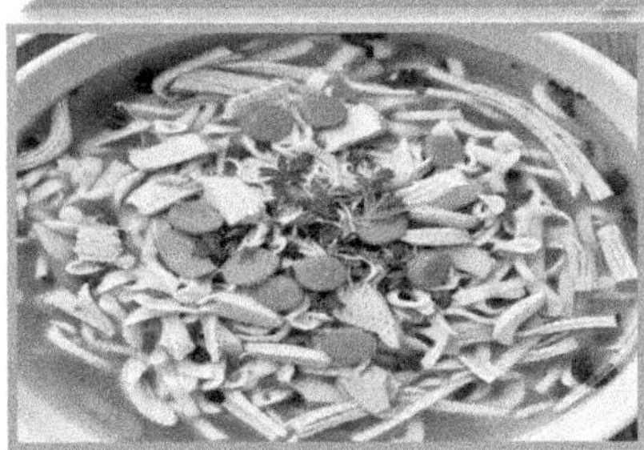

INGREDIENTS

- 2 cups cooked chicken, shredded
- 1 onion, diced
- 2 carrots, diced
- 2 celery stalks, diced
- 3 garlic cloves, minced
- 4 cups chicken broth
- 2 cups egg noodles
- 1 tsp thyme
- Salt and pepper to taste

INSTRUCTIONS

1. Sauté onion, carrots, and celery in a pot until softened.
2. Add garlic and cook for another minute.
3. Pour in chicken broth and bring to a boil.
4. Add noodles, chicken, thyme, salt, and pepper.
5. Simmer for 10 minutes.

Calories: 300, Protein: 25g, Carbs: 30g, Fat: 8g

Tomato Basil Soup

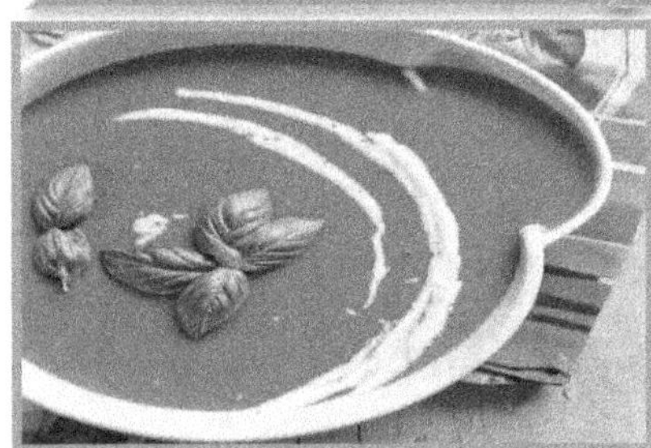

INGREDIENTS

- 2 cans diced tomatoes
- 1 onion, diced
- 3 garlic cloves, minced
- 2 cups vegetable broth
- 1/2 cup heavy cream
- 1/4 cup fresh basil leaves
- Salt and pepper to taste

INSTRUCTIONS

1. Sauté onion and garlic in a pot until softened.
2. Add tomatoes and broth, bring to a boil.
3. Simmer for 15 minutes.
4. Blend the soup until smooth.
5. Stir in heavy cream and basil, season with salt and pepper.

Calories: 220, Protein: 5g, Carbs: 25g, Fat: 10g

Butternut Squash Soup

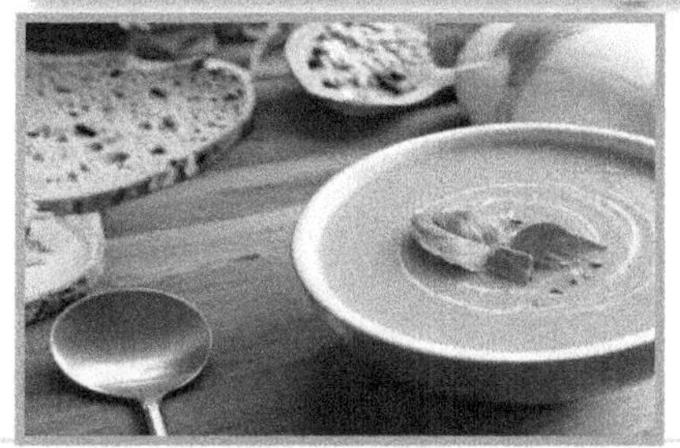

INGREDIENTS

- 1 butternut squash, peeled and cubed
- 1 onion, diced
- 2 carrots, diced
- 2 garlic cloves, minced
- 4 cups vegetable broth
- 1/2 cup coconut milk
- 1 tsp cinnamon
- Salt and pepper to taste

INSTRUCTIONS

1. Sauté onion, carrots, and garlic in a pot until softened.
2. Add squash and broth, bring to a boil.
3. Simmer for 20 minutes.
4. Blend the soup until smooth.
5. Stir in coconut milk and cinnamon, season with salt and pepper.

Calories: 180, Protein: 3g, Carbs: 30g, Fat: 6g

Minestrone Soup

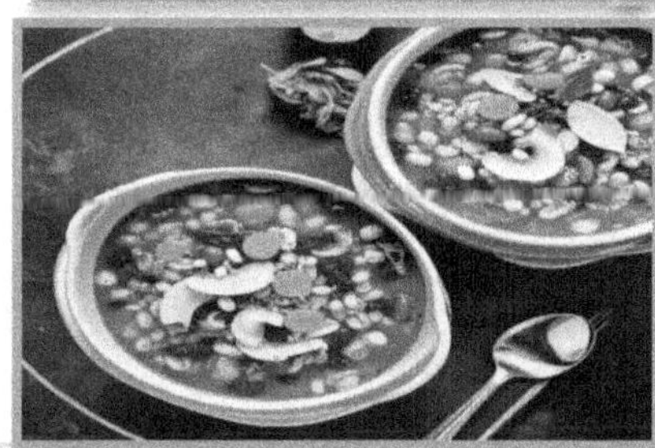

INGREDIENTS

- 1 onion, diced
- 2 carrots, diced
- 2 celery stalks, diced
- 2 garlic cloves, minced
- 1 can diced tomatoes
- 1 can kidney beans, rinsed and drained
- 4 cups vegetable broth
- 1 cup pasta
- 1 zucchini, diced
- 1 tsp Italian seasoning
- Salt and pepper to taste

INSTRUCTIONS

1. Sauté onion, carrots, and celery in a pot until softened.
2. Add garlic and cook for another minute.
3. Add tomatoes, beans, broth, pasta, zucchini, and seasoning.
4. Bring to a boil, then simmer for 20 minutes.

Calories: 250, Protein: 10g, Carbs: 40g, Fat: 5g

Chicken Avocado Wrap

Prep Time: 5 minutes   **Cook Time:** 10 minutes

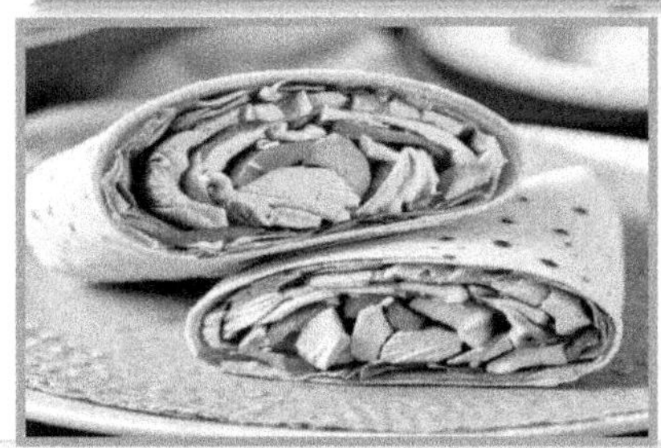

INSTRUCTIONS

1. Lay tortilla flat and spread ranch dressing.
2. Add chicken, avocado, lettuce, and tomatoes.
3. Roll up the tortilla and slice in half.

INGREDIENTS

- 1 whole wheat tortilla
- 1 grilled chicken breast, sliced
- 1/2 avocado, sliced
- 1/4 cup shredded lettuce
- 1/4 cup diced tomatoes
- 1 tbsp ranch dressing

Calories: 350, Protein: 25g, Carbs: 30g, Fat: 15g

Turkey and Hummus Wrap

Prep Time: 5 minutes   **Cook Time:** none minutes

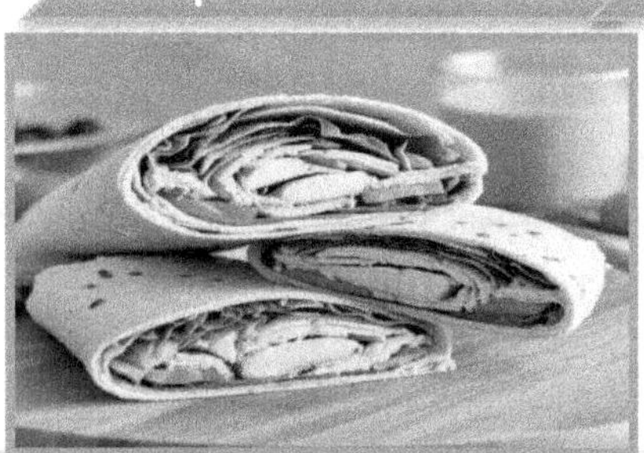

INSTRUCTIONS

1. Lay tortilla flat and spread hummus.
2. Add turkey, carrots, and spinach.
3. Roll up the tortilla and slice in half.

INGREDIENTS

- 1 whole wheat tortilla
- 3 slices turkey breast
- 2 tbsp hummus
- 1/4 cup shredded carrots
- 1/4 cup baby spinach

Calories: 280, Protein: 20g, Carbs: 25g, Fat: 10g

Veggie Wrap

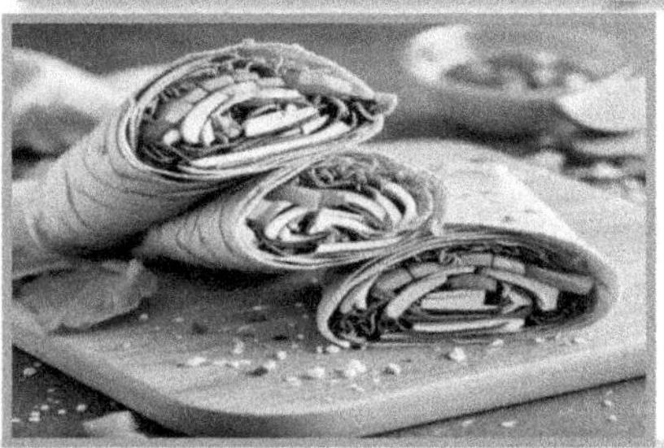

INGREDIENTS

INSTRUCTIONS

1. Lay tortilla flat and spread hummus.
2. Add bell peppers, carrots, and spinach.
3. Roll up the tortilla and slice in half.

- 1 whole wheat tortilla
- 1/4 cup hummus
- 1/4 cup sliced bell peppers
- 1/4 cup shredded carrots
- 1/4 cup baby spinach

Calories: 250, Protein: 7g, Carbs: 30g, Fat: 10g

Tuna Salad Wrap

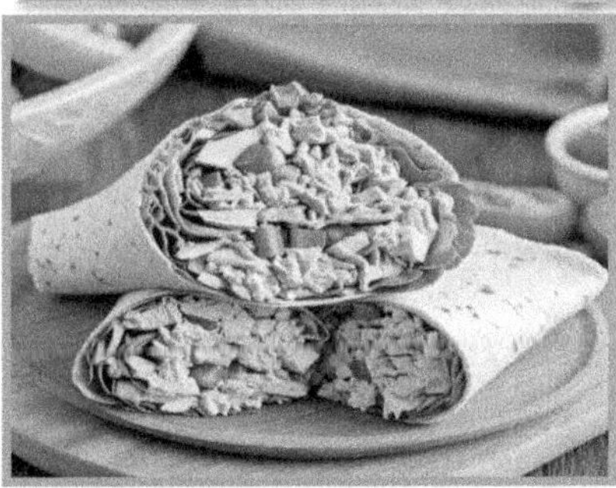

INSTRUCTIONS

1. In a bowl, mix tuna, Greek yogurt, lemon juice, and celery.
2. Lay tortilla flat and add tuna mixture.
3. Top with lettuce, roll up the tortilla, and slice in half.

INGREDIENTS

- 1 whole wheat tortilla
- 1 can tuna, drained
- 2 tbsp Greek yogurt
- 1 tbsp lemon juice
- 1/4 cup diced celery
- 1/4 cup shredded lettuce

Calories: 300, Protein: 25g, Carbs: 25g, Fat: 10g

BBQ Chicken Wrap

Prep Time: 5 minutes   **Cook Time:** 10 minutes

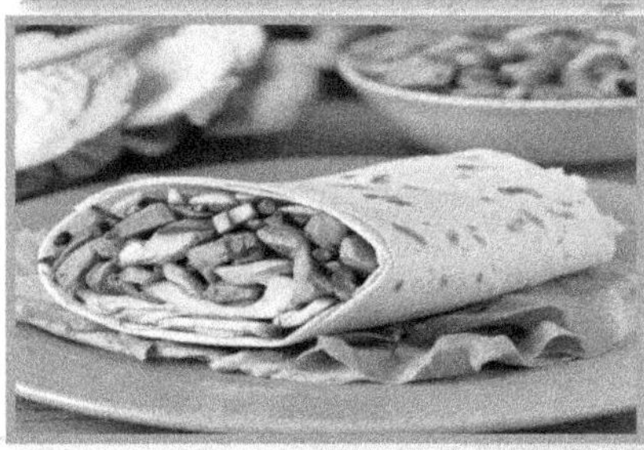

INGREDIENTS

- 1 whole wheat tortilla
- 1 grilled chicken breast, shredded
- 2 tbsp BBQ sauce
- 1/4 cup shredded lettuce
- 1/4 cup shredded cheddar cheese

INSTRUCTIONS

1. Mix shredded chicken with BBQ sauce.
2. Lay tortilla flat and add chicken mixture.
3. Top with lettuce and cheese, roll up the tortilla, and slice in half.

Calories: 350, Protein: 25g, Carbs: 30g, Fat: 12g

Grain Bowls

Mediterranean Quinoa Bowl

Prep Time: 10 minutes   **Cook Time:** 15 minutes

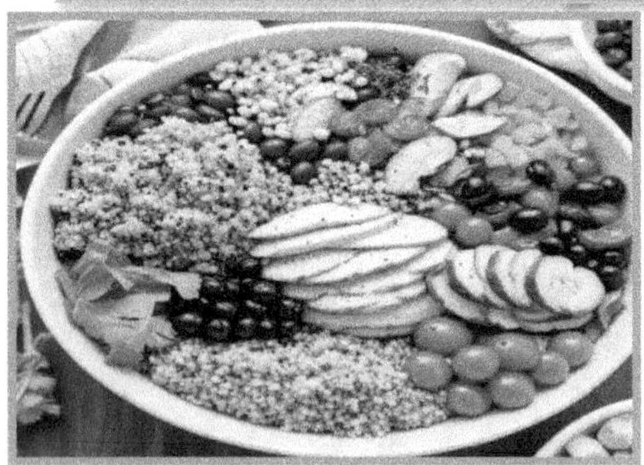

INGREDIENTS

- 1 cup cooked quinoa
- 1/2 cup cherry tomatoes, halved
- 1/4 cup diced cucumber
- 1/4 cup Kalamata olives
- 1/4 cup crumbled feta cheese
- 2 tbsp olive oil
- 1 tbsp lemon juice
- Salt and pepper to taste

INSTRUCTIONS

1. Combine quinoa, tomatoes, cucumber, olives, and feta in a bowl.
2. In a small bowl, whisk together olive oil, lemon juice, salt, and pepper.
3. Pour dressing over the bowl and toss to coat.

Calories: 300, Protein: 10g, Carbs: 30g, Fat: 15g

Teriyaki Chicken Rice Bowl

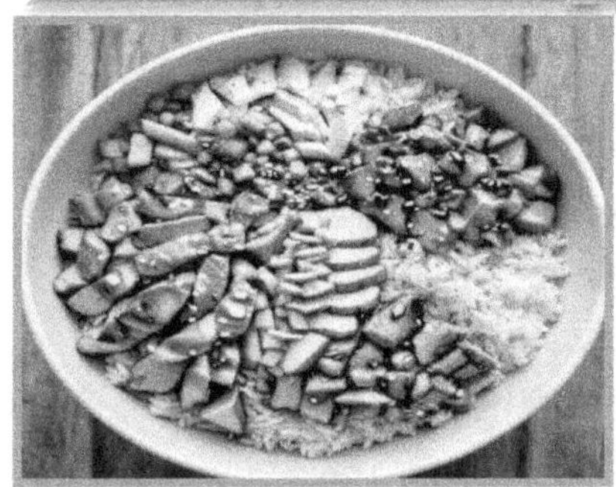

INSTRUCTIONS

1. Place brown rice in a bowl.
2. Top with chicken, broccoli, and carrots.
3. Drizzle with teriyaki sauce and toss gently.

INGREDIENTS

- 1 cup cooked brown rice
- 1 grilled chicken breast, sliced
- 1/2 cup steamed broccoli
- 1/4 cup shredded carrots
- 2 tbsp teriyaki sauce

Calories: 350, Protein: 25g, Carbs: 45g, Fat: 8g

Southwest Black Bean Bowl

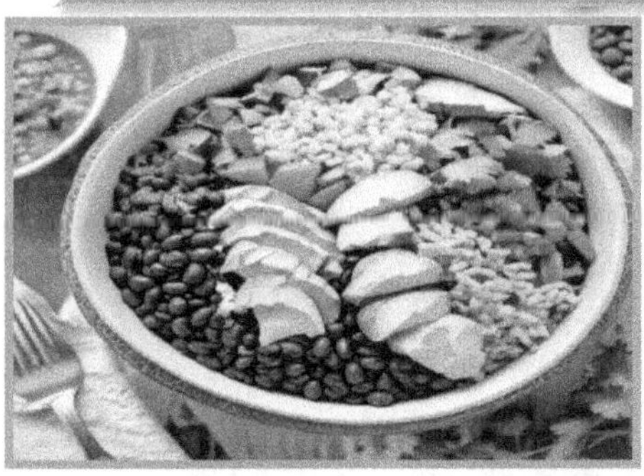

INSTRUCTIONS

1. Place brown rice in a bowl.
2. Top with black beans, corn, tomatoes, and lettuce.
3. Add salsa and sour cream, then toss gently.

INGREDIENTS

- 1 cup cooked brown rice
- 1/2 cup black beans, rinsed and drained
- 1/4 cup corn kernels
- 1/4 cup diced tomatoes
- 1/4 cup shredded lettuce
- 2 tbsp salsa
- 1 tbsp sour cream

Calories: 300, Protein: 10g, Carbs: 50g, Fat: 8g

Buddha Bowl

Prep Time: 10 minutes   **Cook Time:** 20 minutes

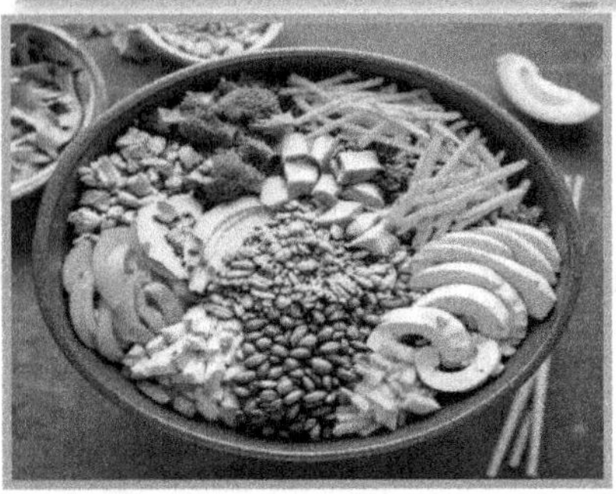

INSTRUCTIONS

1. Place quinoa in a bowl.
2. Top with chickpeas, sweet potatoes, broccoli, and avocado.
3. Drizzle with tahini dressing and toss gently.

INGREDIENTS

- 1 cup cooked quinoa
- 1/4 cup chickpeas, rinsed and drained
- 1/4 cup roasted sweet potatoes
- 1/4 cup steamed broccoli
- 1/4 avocado, sliced
- 2 tbsp tahini dressing

Calories: 350, Protein: 12g, Carbs: 45g, Fat: 15g

Salmon and Brown Rice Bowl

Prep Time: 10 minutes   **Cook Time:** 20 minutes

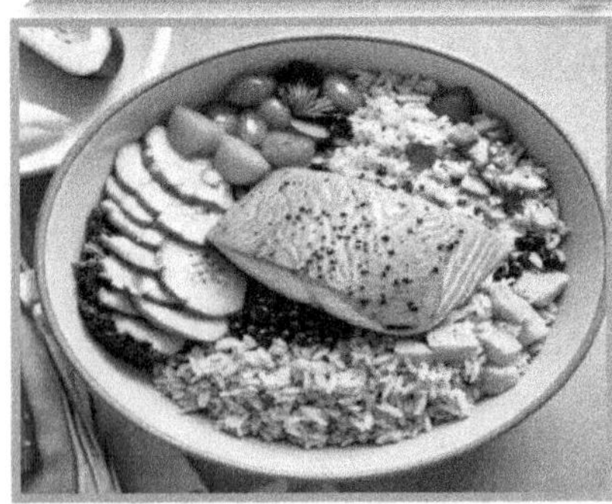

INSTRUCTIONS

1. Place brown rice in a bowl.
2. Top with salmon, asparagus, and cherry tomatoes.
3. Drizzle with lemon dill dressing and toss gently.

INGREDIENTS

- 1 cup cooked brown rice
- 1 grilled salmon fillet, flaked
- 1/4 cup steamed asparagus
- 1/4 cup cherry tomatoes, halved
- 2 tbsp lemon dill dressing

Calories: 400, Protein: 25g, Carbs: 40g, Fat: 15g

Chapter 4: Dinner

"Eating dinner is not a prelude to anything else in the evening. The evening is spent at dinner." This quote by Art Buchwald emphasizes how important a well-thought-out supper is. Portion management and balanced meals are essential while organizing a DASH diet supper as they guarantee dietary requirements are satisfied while limiting salt consumption.

Lean meats, complete grains, healthy fats, and a variety of veggies are usually included in a balanced DASH supper. A platter may include a steamed broccoli portion, a side of quinoa, and a grilled fish fillet, for instance. Vitamins, minerals, and fiber that are vital for general health and digestion may be found in vegetables. Lean proteins, such as those found in chicken, fish, or tofu, keep you full while assisting in tissue growth and repair. Nutrient-dense whole grains, such as brown rice and whole wheat pasta, provide long-lasting energy.

Maintaining a healthy weight and preventing overeating require strict portion management. Smaller servings of nutrient-dense foods are recommended by the DASH diet as opposed to larger servings of high-calorie, low-nutrient meals. To visually control quantities, for example, using smaller dishes may help make it simpler to follow a diet without feeling restricted.

You may make filling and wholesome dinners that follow the DASH diet's guidelines by emphasizing portion management and well-balanced meals, which will eventually improve heart health and general well-being.

Lemon Herb Chicken and Vegetables

Prep Time: 10 minutes   **Cook Time:** 30 minutes

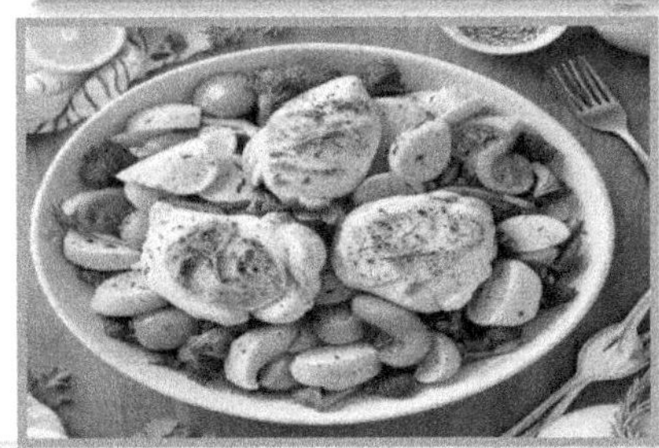

INGREDIENTS

- 4 boneless, skinless chicken breasts
- 1 lb baby potatoes, halved
- 1 lb green beans, trimmed
- 3 tbsp olive oil
- 2 tbsp lemon juice
- 1 tsp garlic powder
- 1 tsp dried oregano
- 1 tsp dried thyme
- Salt and pepper to taste

INSTRUCTIONS

1. Preheat the oven to 400°F (200°C).
2. In a large bowl, combine olive oil, lemon juice, garlic powder, oregano, thyme, salt, and pepper.
3. Add chicken breasts, potatoes, and green beans to the bowl, tossing to coat.
4. Spread everything onto a baking sheet in a single layer.
5. Roast for 25-30 minutes, until chicken is cooked through and vegetables are tender.

Calories: 350, Protein: 30g, Carbs: 30g, Fat: 12g

Teriyaki Beef Stir-Fry

Prep Time: 10 minutes   **Cook Time:** 105minutes

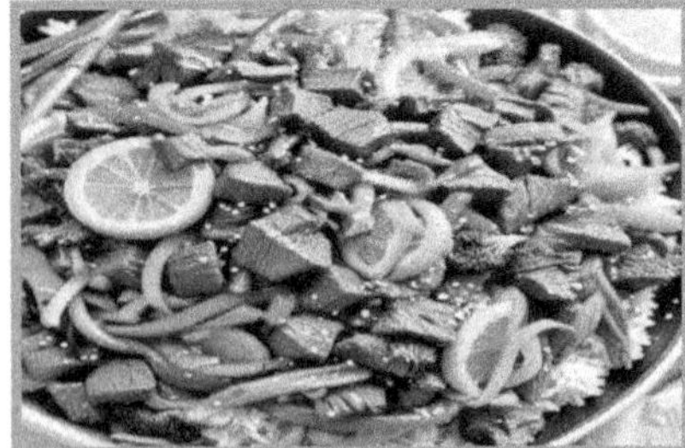

INGREDIENTS

- 1 lb flank steak, thinly sliced
- 1 red bell pepper, sliced
- 1 yellow bell pepper, sliced
- 1 cup broccoli florets
- 1/2 cup teriyaki sauce
- 2 tbsp olive oil
- 2 cloves garlic, minced

INSTRUCTIONS

1. Heat olive oil in a large skillet over medium-high heat.
2. Add garlic and steak slices, cooking until beef is browned, about 5 minutes.
3. Add bell peppers and broccoli, stir-frying for another 5-7 minutes.
4. Pour teriyaki sauce over the mixture, stirring to coat evenly.
5. Cook for an additional 2-3 minutes until sauce thickens.

Calories: 400, Protein: 30g, Carbs: 20g, Fat: 20g

Garlic Shrimp and Asparagus

Prep Time: 10 minutes **Cook Time:** 10 minutes

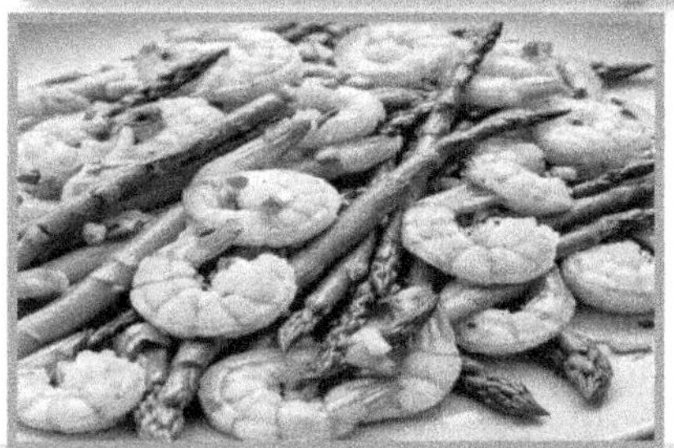

INGREDIENTS

- 1 lb large shrimp, peeled and deveined
- 1 lb asparagus, trimmed and cut into 2-inch pieces
- 3 tbsp olive oil
- 4 cloves garlic, minced
- 1/2 tsp red pepper flakes
- Juice of 1 lemon
- Salt and pepper to taste

INSTRUCTIONS

1. Heat olive oil in a large skillet over medium heat.
2. Add garlic and red pepper flakes, sautéing for 1 minute.
3. Add shrimp and asparagus, cooking until shrimp are pink and asparagus is tender, about 5 minutes.
4. Season with lemon juice, salt, and pepper, and cook for an additional minute.

Calories: 250, Protein: 30g, Carbs: 10g, Fat: 10g

Italian Sausage and Peppers

Prep Time: 10 minutes **Cook Time:** 30 minutes

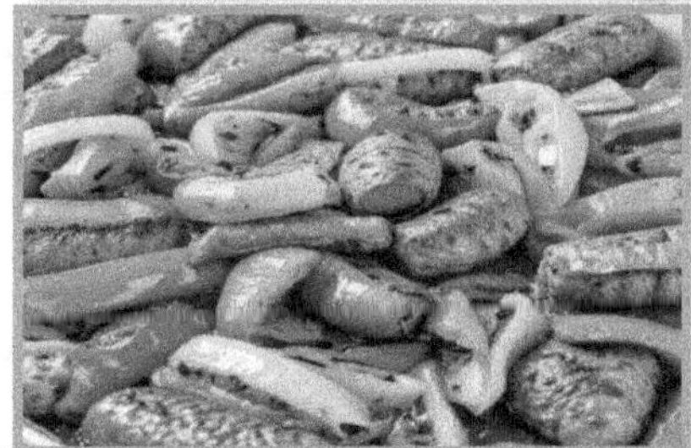

INGREDIENTS

- 4 Italian sausages
- 2 red bell peppers, sliced
- 2 yellow bell peppers, sliced
- 1 large onion, sliced
- 2 tbsp olive oil
- 1 tsp Italian seasoning
- Salt and pepper to taste
-

INSTRUCTIONS

1. Preheat the oven to 400°F (200°C).
2. In a large bowl, toss bell peppers and onion with olive oil, Italian seasoning, salt, and pepper.
3. Spread vegetables onto a baking sheet and top with sausages.
4. Roast for 25-30 minutes, until sausages are cooked through and vegetables are tender.

Calories: 350, Protein: 20g, Carbs: 15g, Fat: 25g

Balsamic Chicken and Vegetables

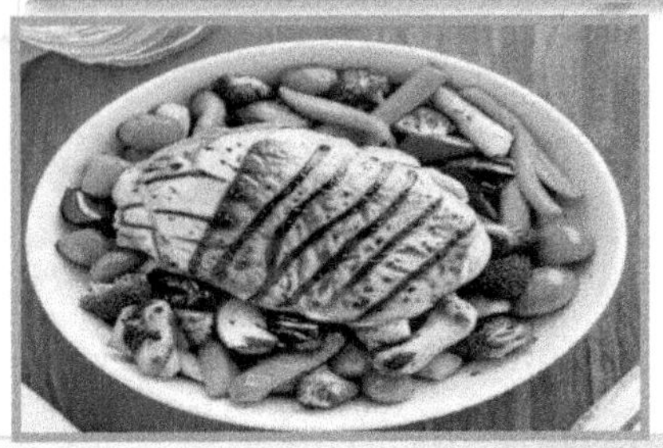

INGREDIENTS

- 4 boneless, skinless chicken thighs
- 1 lb baby potatoes, halved
- 1 lb Brussels sprouts, halved
- 3 tbsp balsamic vinegar
- 3 tbsp olive oil
- 1 tsp garlic powder
- 1 tsp dried rosemary
- Salt and pepper to taste

INSTRUCTIONS

1. Preheat the oven to 400°F (200°C).
2. In a large bowl, combine balsamic vinegar, olive oil, garlic powder, rosemary, salt, and pepper.
3. Add chicken thighs, potatoes, and Brussels sprouts to the bowl, tossing to coat.
4. Spread everything onto a baking sheet in a single layer.
5. Roast for 25-30 minutes, until chicken is cooked through and vegetables are tender.

Calories: 400, Protein: 25g, Carbs: 35g, Fat: 20g

Comfort Classics

Chicken Pot Pie

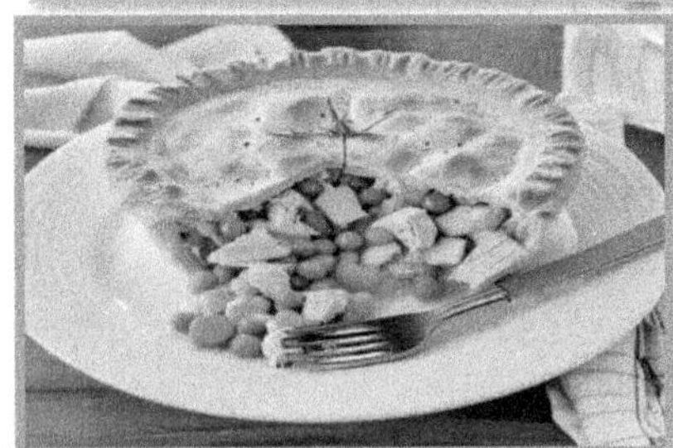

INGREDIENTS

- 1 lb chicken breast, cooked and diced
- 1 cup frozen peas and carrots
- 1/2 cup frozen corn
- 1/2 cup diced potatoes
- 1/4 cup butter
- 1/4 cup flour
- 2 cups chicken broth
- 1 cup milk
- Salt and pepper to taste
- 1 refrigerated pie crust

INSTRUCTIONS

1. Preheat the oven to 425°F (220°C).
2. In a large pot, melt butter over medium heat. Stir in flour until well combined.
3. Gradually add chicken broth and milk, stirring until thickened.
4. Add chicken, peas, carrots, corn, potatoes, salt, and pepper. Cook for 5 minutes.
5. Pour mixture into a pie dish and cover with pie crust, sealing the edges.
6. Bake for 30 minutes, until crust is golden brown.

Calories: 450, Protein: 25g, Carbs: 40g, Fat: 20g

Beef Stroganoff

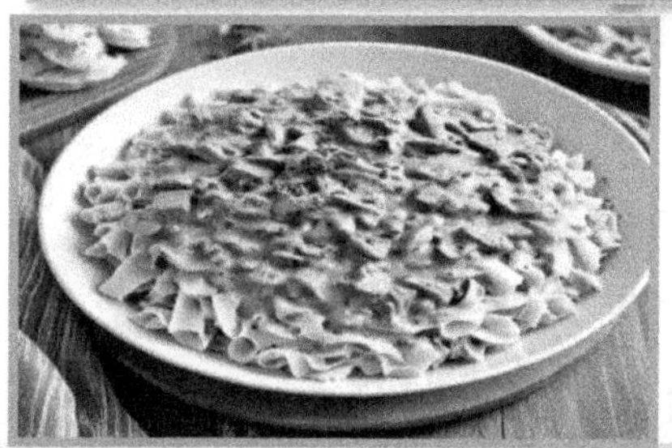

INGREDIENTS

- 1 lb beef sirloin, thinly sliced
- 1 onion, diced
- 1 cup mushrooms, sliced
- 2 cloves garlic, minced
- 2 tbsp olive oil
- 1 cup beef broth
- 1 cup sour cream
- 2 tbsp flour
- Salt and pepper to taste
- Egg noodles, for serving

INSTRUCTIONS

1. Heat olive oil in a large skillet over medium-high heat.
2. Add beef and cook until browned. Remove and set aside.
3. In the same skillet, sauté onion, mushrooms, and garlic until tender.
4. Stir in flour, then gradually add beef broth and sour cream, stirring until thickened.
5. Return beef to the skillet, cooking for an additional 5 minutes.
6. Serve over cooked egg noodles.

Calories: 500, Protein: 30g, Carbs: 45g, Fat: 20g

Shepherd's Pie

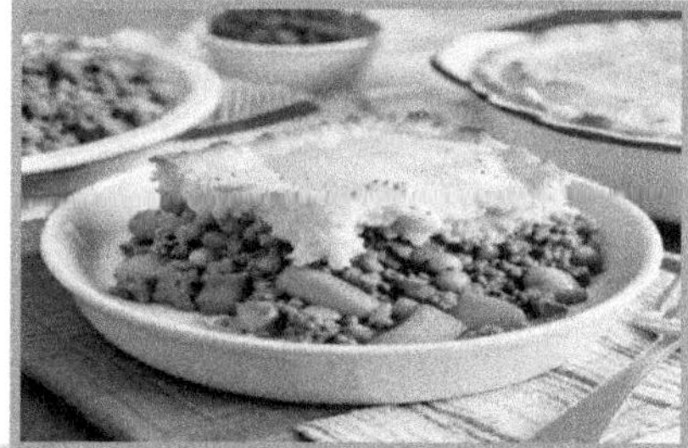

INGREDIENTS

- 1 lb ground lamb or beef
- 1 onion, diced
- 2 carrots, diced
- 1 cup frozen peas
- 2 tbsp tomato paste
- 1 cup beef broth
- 4 cups mashed potatoes
- 2 tbsp olive oil
- Salt and pepper to taste

INSTRUCTIONS

1. Preheat the oven to 400°F (200°C).
2. Heat olive oil in a large skillet over medium heat. Add ground meat, cooking until browned.
3. Add onion, carrots, and peas, cooking until tender. Stir in tomato paste and beef broth.
4. Pour mixture into a baking dish and top with mashed potatoes.
5. Bake for 25-30 minutes, until potatoes are golden brown.

Calories: 400, Protein: 25g, Carbs: 45g, Fat: 15g

Meatloaf

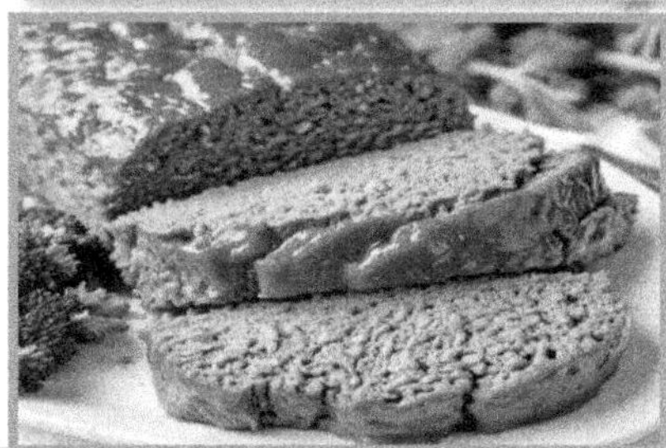

INGREDIENTS

- 1 lb ground beef
- 1 onion, finely chopped
- 1/2 cup breadcrumbs
- 1/2 cup milk
- 1 egg
- 1/4 cup ketchup
- 2 tbsp Worcestershire sauce
- Salt and pepper to taste

INSTRUCTIONS

1. Preheat the oven to 375°F (190°C).
2. In a large bowl, combine all ingredients and mix well.
3. Shape mixture into a loaf and place in a baking dish.
4. Bake for 45-50 minutes, until cooked through.

Calories: 350, Protein: 20g, Carbs: 20g, Fat: 20g

Seafood Delights

Lemon Herb Baked Salmon

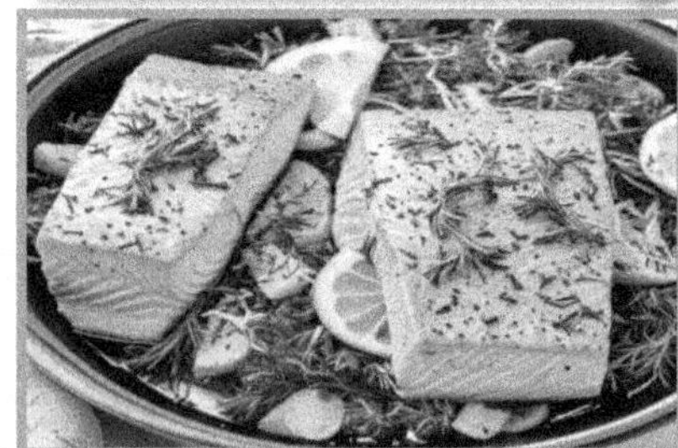

INGREDIENTS

- 4 salmon fillets
- 2 lemons, thinly sliced
- 2 tbsp olive oil
- 2 tbsp fresh dill, chopped
- 2 tbsp fresh parsley, chopped
- Salt and pepper to taste

INSTRUCTIONS

1. Preheat the oven to 375°F (190°C).
2. Place salmon fillets on a baking sheet lined with parchment paper.
3. Drizzle olive oil over the fillets, and season with salt and pepper.
4. Top with lemon slices, dill, and parsley.
5. Bake for 20-25 minutes, until the salmon is cooked through.

Calories: 300, Protein: 25g, Carbs: 5g, Fat: 20g

Garlic Shrimp Stir-Fry

Prep Time: 10 minutes   **Cook Time:** 15 minutes

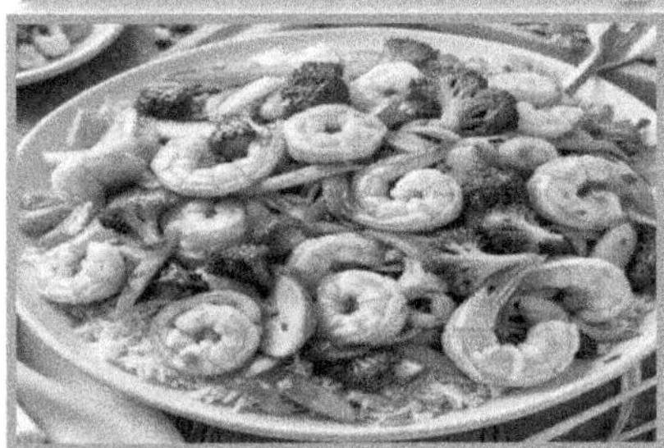

INGREDIENTS

- 1 lb large shrimp, peeled and deveined
- 2 cups broccoli florets
- 1 red bell pepper, sliced
- 1 yellow bell pepper, sliced
- 3 cloves garlic, minced
- 2 tbsp olive oil
- 1 tbsp soy sauce
- 1 tbsp lemon juice
- Salt and pepper to taste

INSTRUCTIONS

1. Heat olive oil in a large skillet over medium-high heat.
2. Add garlic and cook until fragrant, about 1 minute.
3. Add shrimp and cook until pink, about 3-4 minutes. Remove from skillet and set aside.
4. Add broccoli and bell peppers to the skillet and cook until tender-crisp, about 5-7 minutes.
5. Return shrimp to the skillet, add soy sauce and lemon juice, and stir to combine.
6. Serve hot.

Calories: 250, Protein: 25g, Carbs: 10g, Fat: 10g

Grilled Tuna Steaks with Mango Salsa

Prep Time: 15 minutes   **Cook Time:** 10 minutes

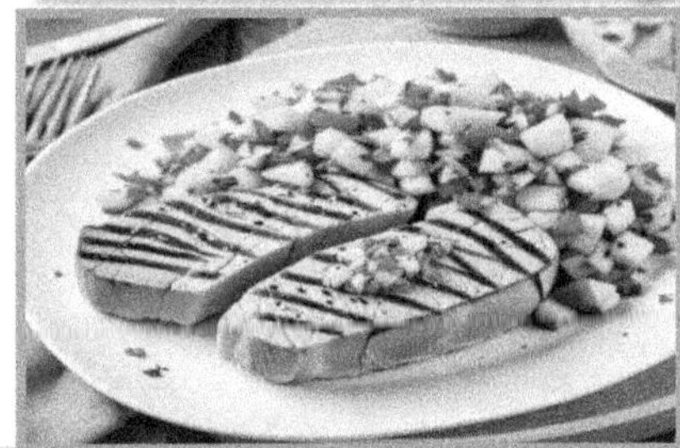

INGREDIENTS

- 4 tuna steaks
- 2 tbsp olive oil
- Salt and pepper to taste
- 1 mango, diced
- 1/4 cup red onion, finely chopped
- 1/4 cup fresh cilantro, chopped
- 1 lime, juiced
- 1 jalapeño, seeded and minced

INSTRUCTIONS

1. Preheat the grill to medium-high heat.
2. Brush tuna steaks with olive oil and season with salt and pepper.
3. Grill tuna steaks for 4-5 minutes per side, until desired doneness.
4. In a bowl, combine mango, red onion, cilantro, lime juice, and jalapeño to make salsa.
5. Serve grilled tuna steaks topped with mango salsa.

Calories: 350, Protein: 30g, Carbs: 15g, Fat: 15g

Baked Cod with Tomatoes and Olives

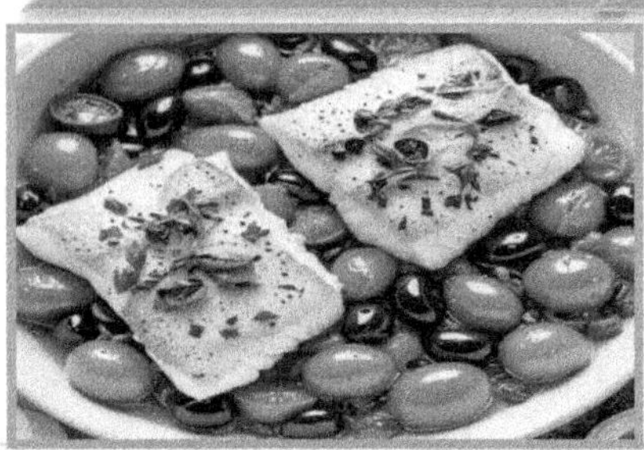

INSTRUCTIONS

1. Preheat the oven to 400°F (200°C).
2. Place cod fillets in a baking dish and season with salt and pepper.
3. In a bowl, combine cherry tomatoes, olives, garlic, olive oil, and basil.
4. Pour tomato mixture over cod fillets.
5. Bake for 20-25 minutes, until the cod is cooked through.

INGREDIENTS

- 4 cod fillets
- 1 pint cherry tomatoes, halved
- 1/2 cup Kalamata olives, sliced
- 2 cloves garlic, minced
- 2 tbsp olive oil
- 1 tbsp fresh basil, chopped
- Salt and pepper to taste

Calories: 250, Protein: 30g, Carbs: 10g, Fat: 10g

Shrimp and Avocado Salad

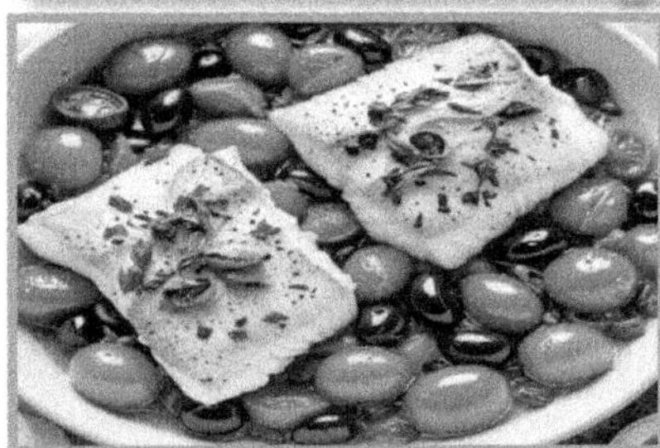

INSTRUCTIONS

1. Heat olive oil in a skillet over medium-high heat.
2. Add shrimp and cook until pink, about 3-4 minutes. Remove from heat and let cool.
3. In a large bowl, combine shrimp, avocados, cucumber, red onion, and cilantro.
4. Drizzle with lime juice and olive oil, and season with salt and pepper.
5. Toss to combine and serve chilled.

INGREDIENTS

- 1 lb large shrimp, peeled and deveined
- 2 avocados, diced
- 1 cucumber, diced
- 1/4 cup red onion, finely chopped
- 1/4 cup fresh cilantro, chopped
- 1 lime, juiced
- 2 tbsp olive oil
- Salt and pepper to taste

Calories: 300. Protein: 25g. Carbs: 15g. Fat: 20g

Variations: *Add cherry tomatoes or use lemon juice instead of lime juice.*

Sweet Potato and Black Bean Chili

Prep Time: 15 minutes **Cook Time:** 25 minutes

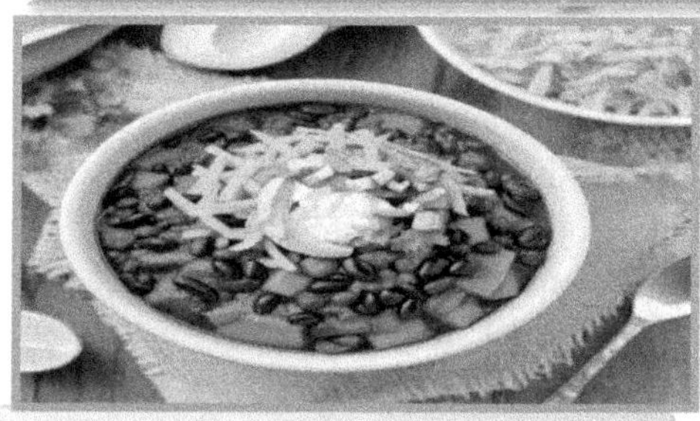

INSTRUCTIONS

1. Heat olive oil in a large pot over medium heat.
2. Add onion and garlic, sautéing until translucent.
3. Stir in sweet potatoes, black beans, diced tomatoes, chili powder, cumin, salt, and pepper.
4. Add enough water to cover ingredients, bring to a boil, then reduce heat and simmer for 20-25 minutes, until sweet potatoes are tender.
5. Serve hot, garnished with fresh cilantro.

INGREDIENTS

- 2 sweet potatoes, peeled and diced
- 1 can black beans, drained and rinsed
- 1 can diced tomatoes
- 1 onion, diced
- 2 cloves garlic, minced
- 1 tbsp chili powder
- 1 tsp cumin
- Salt and pepper to taste
- Fresh cilantro for garnish

Calories: 350, Protein: 10g, Carbs: 65g, Fat: 5g

Caprese Stuffed Portobello Mushrooms

Prep Time: 10 minutes **Cook Time:** 20 minutes

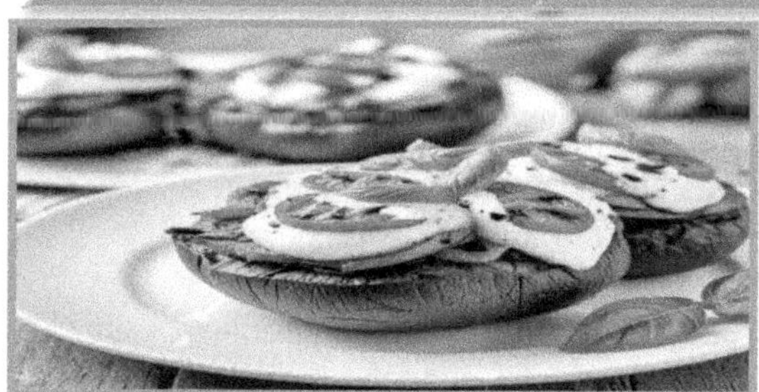

INSTRUCTIONS

1. Preheat the oven to 400°F (200°C).
2. In a bowl, combine cherry tomatoes, mozzarella, basil, balsamic vinegar, olive oil, salt, and pepper.
3. Spoon mixture into portobello mushrooms.
4. Place stuffed mushrooms on a baking sheet and bake for 15-20 minutes, until mushrooms are tender and cheese is melted.

INGREDIENTS

- 4 portobello mushrooms, stems removed
- 1 cup cherry tomatoes, halved
- 1 cup fresh mozzarella, diced
- 1/2 cup fresh basil leaves, chopped
- 2 tbsp balsamic vinegar
- 2 tbsp olive oil
- Salt and pepper to taste

Calories: 250, Protein: 15g, Carbs: 10g, Fat: 15g

Veggie Stir-Fry with Tofu

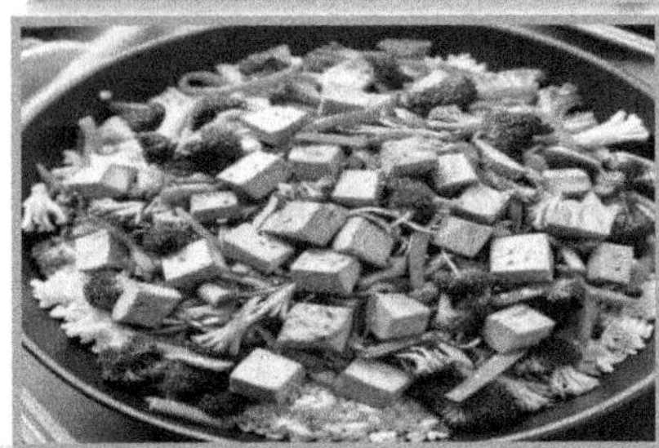

INGREDIENTS

- 1 block firm tofu, drained and cubed
- 2 cups broccoli florets
- 1 red bell pepper, sliced
- 1 yellow bell pepper, sliced
- 1 cup snap peas
- 1/4 cup soy sauce
- 2 tbsp hoisin sauce
- 2 tbsp olive oil
- 2 cloves garlic, minced
- 1 tsp ginger, minced
- Sesame seeds for garnish

INSTRUCTIONS

1. Heat olive oil in a large skillet or wok over medium-high heat.
2. Add tofu cubes and cook until golden brown on all sides, about 5-7 minutes. Remove from skillet and set aside.
3. In the same skillet, add garlic and ginger, sautéing until fragrant, about 1 minute.
4. Add broccoli, bell peppers, and snap peas, stir-frying until vegetables are tender-crisp, about 5 minutes.
5. Return tofu to the skillet, add soy sauce and hoisin sauce, stirring until heated through and well coated.
6. Serve hot, garnished with sesame seeds.

Calories: 300, Protein: 20g, Carbs: 25g, Fat: 15g

Spinach and Ricotta Stuffed Shells

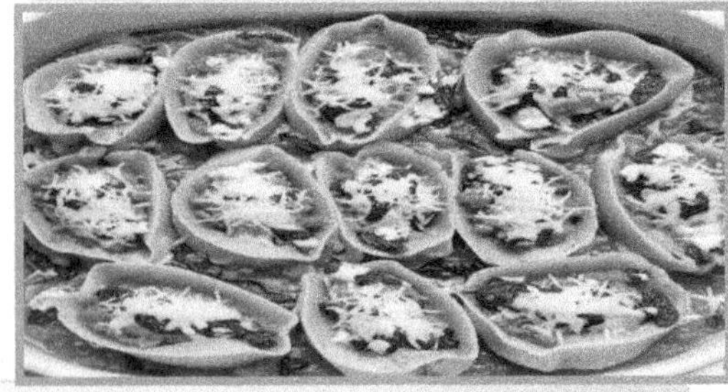

INGREDIENTS

- 1 box jumbo pasta shells
- 2 cups ricotta cheese
- 1 cup shredded mozzarella cheese
- 1 cup grated Parmesan cheese
- 2 cups spinach, chopped
- 1 egg
- 2 cups marinara sauce
- Salt and pepper to taste
- Fresh basil for garnish

INSTRUCTIONS

1. Preheat the oven to 375°F (190°C).
2. Cook pasta shells according to package instructions. Drain and set aside.
3. In a bowl, combine ricotta cheese, mozzarella cheese, Parmesan cheese, spinach, egg, salt, and pepper.
4. Stuff cooked shells with ricotta mixture and place in a baking dish.
5. Pour marinara sauce over shells, covering evenly.
6. Bake for 25-30 minutes, until sauce is bubbly and cheese is melted.
7. Serve hot, garnished with fresh basil.

Calories: 450, Protein: 25g, Carbs: 50g, Fat: 20g

Mediterranean Chickpea Salad

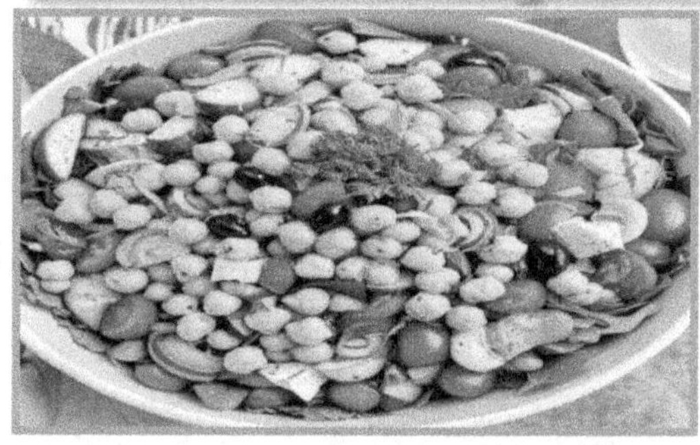

INSTRUCTIONS

1. In a large bowl, combine chickpeas, cucumber, cherry tomatoes, olives, red onion, and feta cheese.
2. In a small bowl, whisk together olive oil, red wine vinegar, oregano, salt, and pepper.
3. Pour dressing over chickpea mixture, tossing until well coated.
4. Serve chilled or at room temperature.

INGREDIENTS

- 2 cans chickpeas, drained and rinsed
- 1 cucumber, diced
- 1 pint cherry tomatoes, halved
- 1/2 cup Kalamata olives, sliced
- 1/4 cup red onion, thinly sliced
- 1/2 cup crumbled feta cheese
- 2 tbsp olive oil
- 2 tbsp red wine vinegar
- 1 tsp dried oregano
- Salt and pepper to taste

Calories: 350, Protein: 15g, Carbs: 45g, Fat: 15g

Chapter 5: Snacks and Sides

Snacking healthily may have a big influence on your energy levels and general health, according to American Heart Association studies. Snacks are an important part of the DASH diet because they help keep blood sugar levels in check and provide key nutrients in between meals. Simple but healthy snack options include almond butter on apple slices, hummus on vegetable sticks, and Greek yogurt with berries. These snacks are great for sating your appetite since they're high in fiber, protein, and good fats. They're also tasty.

You may maintain your nutritional objectives by including DASH-friendly snacks in your routine. Greek yogurt, for instance, is high in protein and probiotics, which help to maintain gut health and keep you feeling full. Hummus-topped veggie sticks make a crisp, filling snack that's rich in fiber and important vitamins. In the meanwhile, apple slices with almond butter provide a savory and sweet combo that is filling and healthy.

Snacking healthily also lessens the chance of overindulging during meals. Selecting foods high in nutrients can help you control your weight, strengthen your heart, and have steady energy levels all day. The DASH diet may be easily followed and made to seem like a fun part of your daily routine with the correct snacks.

Greek Yogurt with Honey and Walnuts

Prep Time: 5 minutes   **Cook Time:** 0 minutes

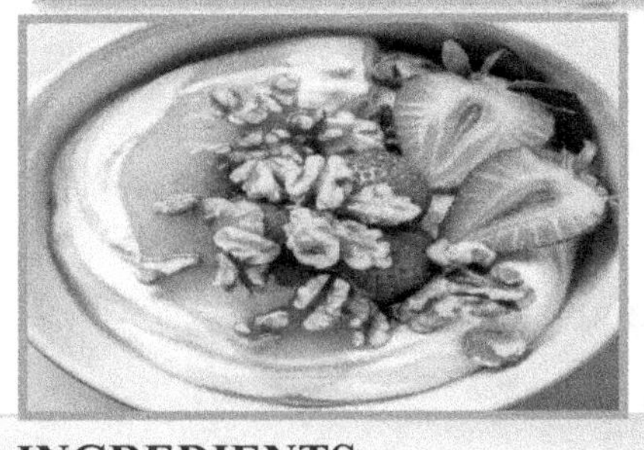

INSTRUCTIONS

1. Spoon Greek yogurt into a bowl.
2. Drizzle with honey.
3. Top with chopped walnuts.

INGREDIENTS

- 1 cup Greek yogurt
- 1 tbsp honey
- 2 tbsp chopped walnuts

Calories: 200, Protein: 15g, Carbs: 20g, Fat: 8g

Almond Butter Banana Bites

Prep Time: 5 minutes   **Cook Time:** 0 minutes

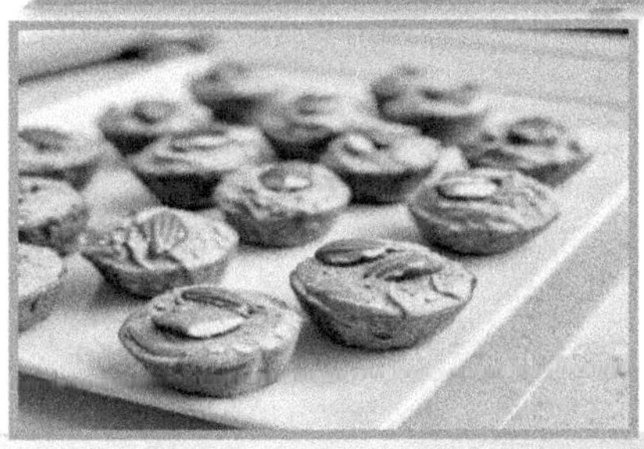

INSTRUCTIONS

1. Spread almond butter on each banana slice.
2. Sprinkle with chia seeds.

INGREDIENTS

- 1 banana, sliced
- 2 tbsp almond butter
- 1 tbsp chia seeds

Calories: 150, Protein: 3g, Carbs: 20g, Fat: 8g

Cottage Cheese with Pineapple

Prep Time: 5 minutes   **Cook Time:** 0 minutes

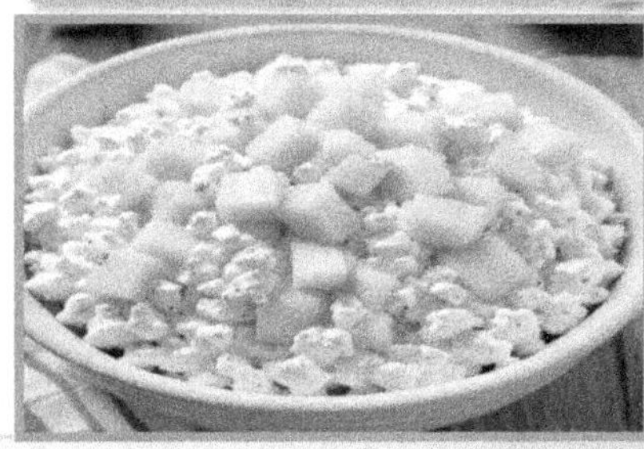

INSTRUCTIONS

1. Spoon cottage cheese into a bowl.
2. Top with pineapple chunks and shredded coconut.

INGREDIENTS

- 1 cup cottage cheese
- 1/2 cup pineapple chunks
- 1 tbsp shredded coconut

Calories: 180, Protein: 15g, Carbs: 20g, Fat: 5g

Veggie Sticks with Hummus

Prep Time: 10 minutes   **Cook Time:** 0 minutes

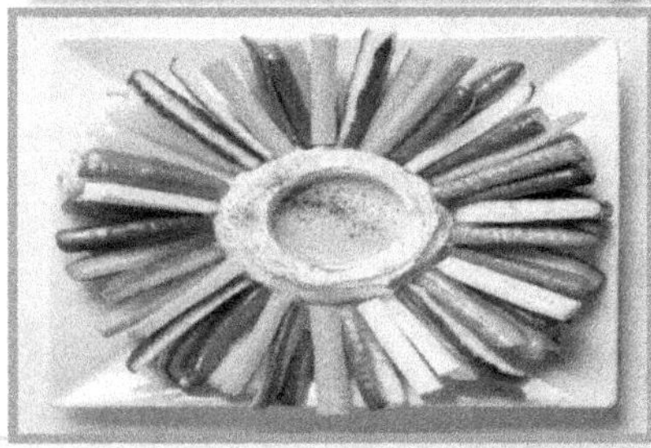

INSTRUCTIONS

1. Arrange veggie sticks on a plate.
2. Serve with hummus for dipping.

INGREDIENTS

- 1 cup hummus
- 1 carrot, cut into sticks
- 1 cucumber, cut into sticks
- 1 red bell pepper, cut into sticks

Calories: 150, Protein: 4g, Carbs: 20g, Fat: 6g

Apple Slices with Almond Butter

Prep Time: 5 minutes   **Cook Time:** 0 minutes

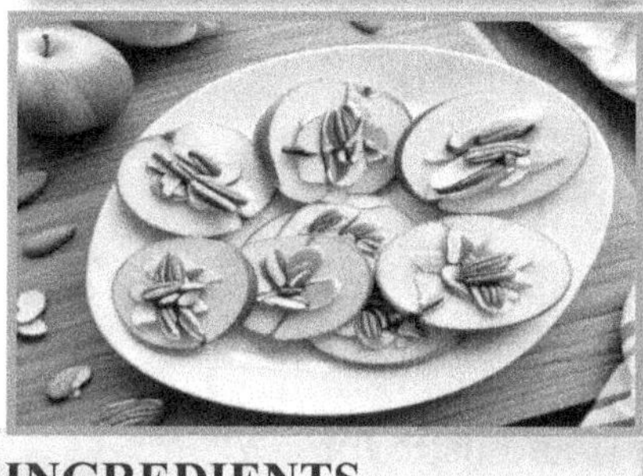

INSTRUCTIONS

1. Spread almond butter on apple slices.

INGREDIENTS

- 1 apple, sliced
- 2 tbsp almond butter

Calories: 150, Protein: 2g, Carbs: 22g, Fat: 8g

Crunchy Bites

Roasted Chickpeas

Prep Time: 10 minutes   **Cook Time:** 30 minutes

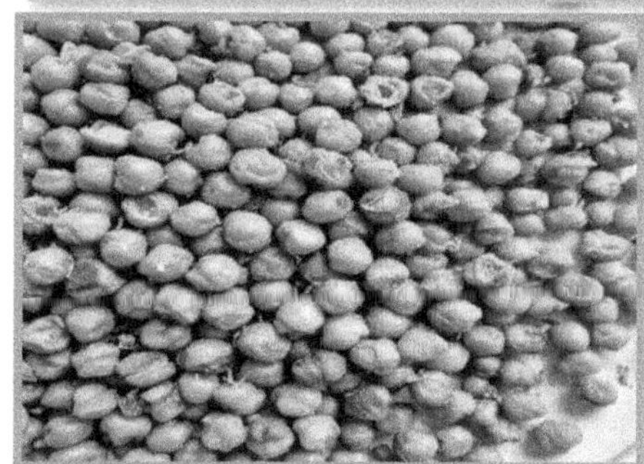

INSTRUCTIONS

1. Preheat oven to 400°F (200°C).
2. Toss chickpeas with olive oil, smoked paprika, garlic powder, salt, and pepper.
3. Spread on a baking sheet and roast for 25-30 minutes, until crispy.

INGREDIENTS

- 1 can chickpeas, drained and rinsed
- 1 tbsp olive oil
- 1 tsp smoked paprika
- 1/2 tsp garlic powder
- Salt and pepper to taste

Calories: 120, Protein: 5g, Carbs: 20g, Fat: 4g

Kale Chips

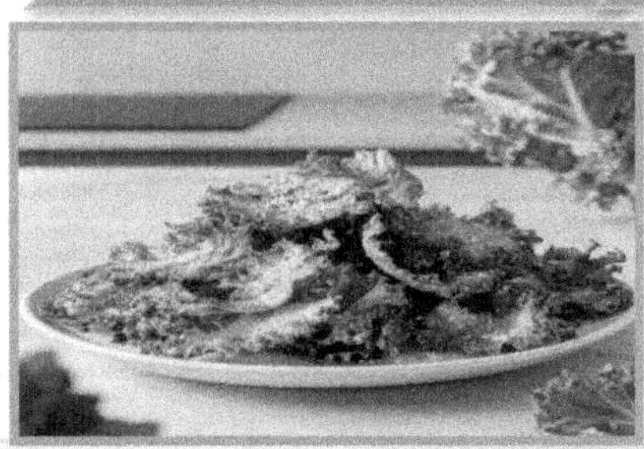

INSTRUCTIONS

1. Preheat oven to 350°F (175°C).
2. Remove kale leaves from stems and tear into bite-sized pieces.
3. Toss with olive oil and salt.
4. Spread on a baking sheet and bake for 10-15 minutes, until crispy.

INGREDIENTS

- 1 bunch kale, washed and dried
- 1 tbsp olive oil
- Salt to taste

Calories: 50, Protein: 2g, Carbs: 8g, Fat: 3g

Spiced Nuts

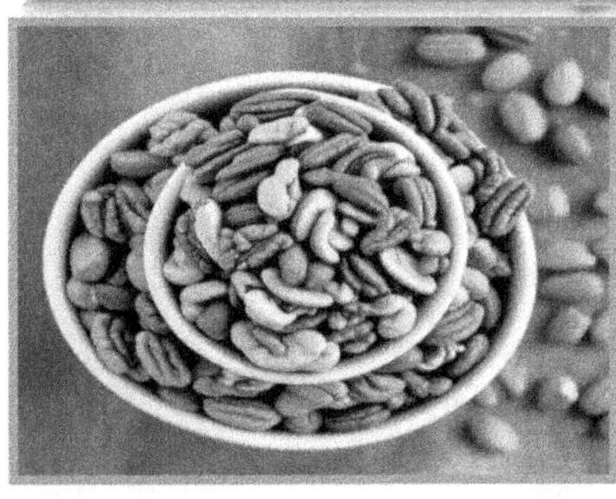

INSTRUCTIONS

1. Preheat oven to 350°F (175°C).
2. Toss nuts with olive oil and spices.
3. Spread on a baking sheet and bake for 10-15 minutes, until fragrant.

INGREDIENTS

- 1 cup mixed nuts (almonds, cashews, walnuts)
- 1 tbsp olive oil
- 1 tsp chili powder
- 1/2 tsp cumin
- 1/2 tsp paprika
- Salt to taste

Calories: 200, Protein: 5g, Carbs: 6g, Fat: 18g

Baked Zucchini Fries

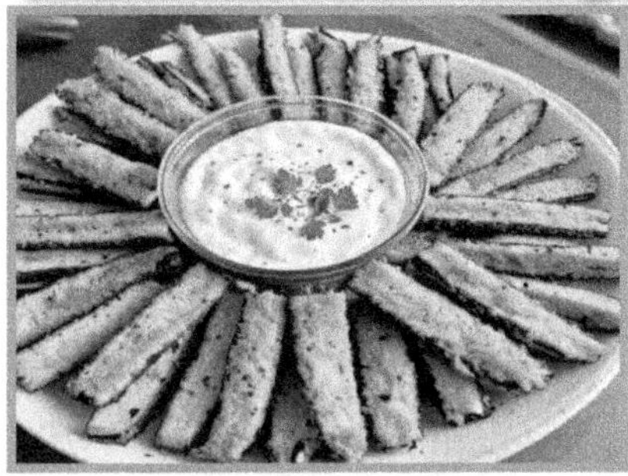

INSTRUCTIONS

1. Preheat oven to 425°F (220°C).
2. Mix breadcrumbs, Parmesan cheese, and Italian seasoning in a bowl.
3. Dip zucchini sticks in egg, then coat with breadcrumb mixture.
4. Place on a baking sheet and bake for 20-25 minutes, until golden brown.

INGREDIENTS

- 2 zucchinis, cut into sticks
- 1/2 cup whole wheat breadcrumbs
- 1/4 cup grated Parmesan cheese
- 1 tsp Italian seasoning
- 1 egg, beaten

Calories: 150, Protein: 6g, Carbs: 20g, Fat: 6g

Carrot and Cucumber Rolls

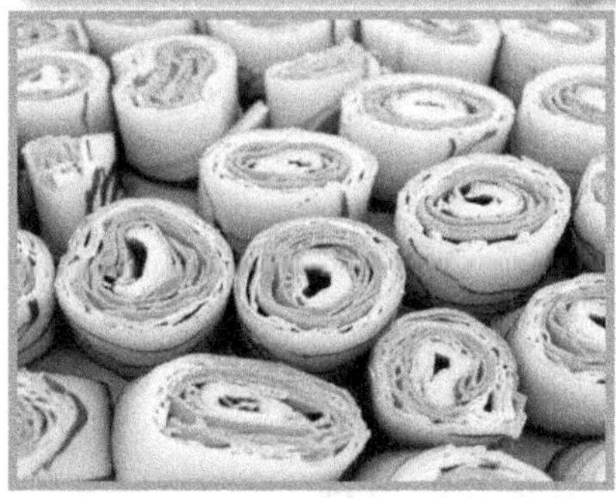

INSTRUCTIONS

1. Spread hummus on each vegetable slice.
2. Sprinkle with fresh herbs.
3. Roll up and secure with a toothpick.

INGREDIENTS

- 1 carrot, thinly sliced
- 1 cucumber, thinly sliced
- 1/2 cup hummus
- 1/4 cup chopped fresh herbs (parsley, cilantro, mint)

Calories: 80, Protein: 2g, Carbs: 12g, Fat: 3g

Tomato and Cucumber Salad

Prep Time: 10 minutes   **Cook Time:** 0 minutes

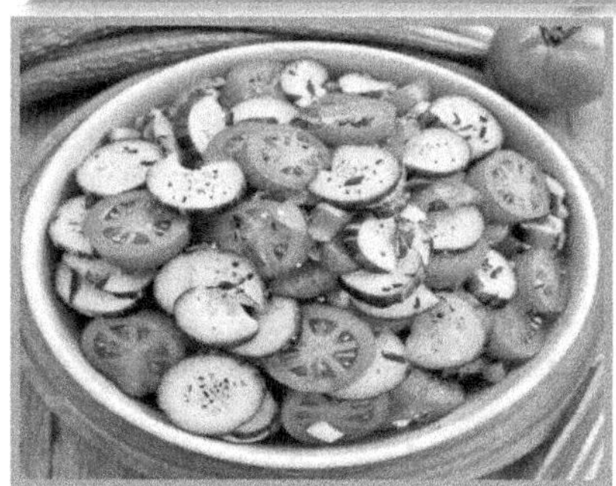

INSTRUCTIONS

1. Combine tomatoes, cucumber, and red onion in a bowl.
2. Drizzle with olive oil and vinegar.
3. Season with salt and pepper, and toss to combine.

INGREDIENTS

- 2 cups cherry tomatoes, halved
- 1 cucumber, diced
- 1/4 red onion, thinly sliced
- 2 tbsp olive oil
- 1 tbsp red wine vinegar
- Salt and pepper to taste

Calories: 120, Protein: 2g, Carbs: 10g, Fat: 8g

Quinoa Salad

Prep Time: 10 minutes   **Cook Time:** 0 minutes

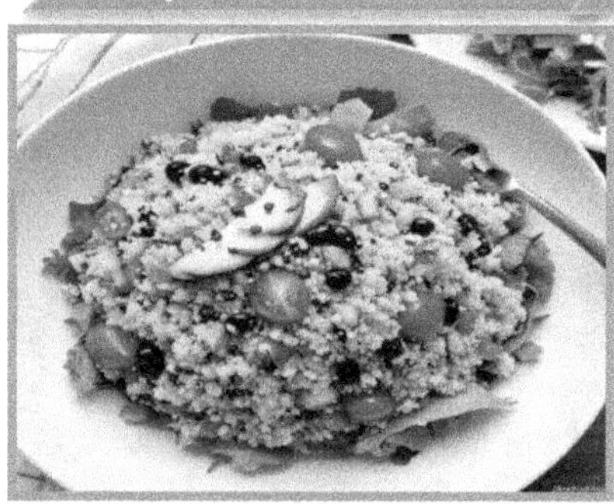

INSTRUCTIONS

1. In a bowl, combine quinoa, bell peppers, and parsley.
2. Drizzle with olive oil and lemon juice.
3. Season with salt and pepper, and toss to combine.

INGREDIENTS

- 1 cup cooked quinoa
- 1/2 cup diced bell peppers
- 1/4 cup chopped fresh parsley
- 2 tbsp olive oil
- 1 tbsp lemon juice
- Salt and pepper to taste

Calories: 150, Protein: 5g, Carbs: 20g, Fat: 6g

Fruit Salad

Prep Time: 10 minutes   **Cook Time:** 0 minutes

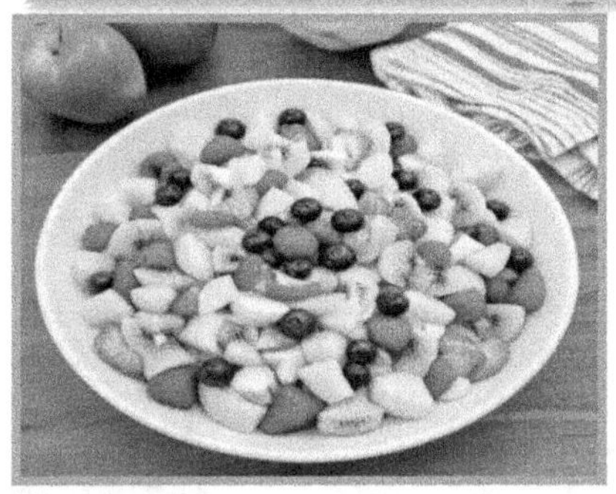

INSTRUCTIONS

1. In a large bowl, combine pineapple, watermelon, and grapes.
2. Drizzle with honey and lime juice, and toss to combine.

INGREDIENTS

- 1 cup diced pineapple
- 1 cup diced watermelon
- 1 cup halved grapes
- 1 tbsp honey
- 1 tbsp lime juice

Calories: 100, Protein: 1g, Carbs: 25g, Fat: 0g

Steamed Green Beans with Almonds

Prep Time: 5 minutes   **Cook Time:** 7 minutes

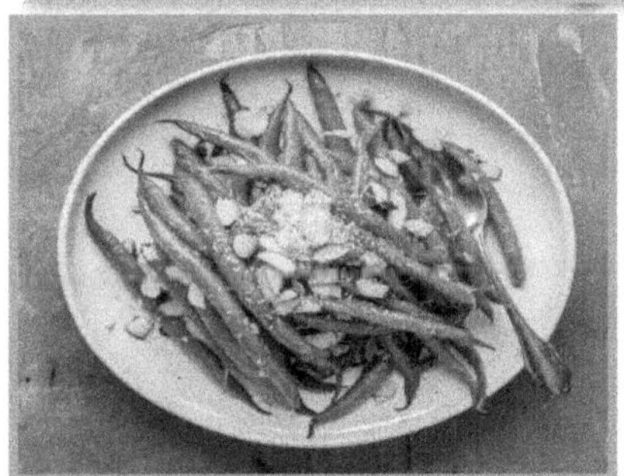

INSTRUCTIONS

1. Steam green beans until tender, about 5-7 minutes.
2. Toss with olive oil, almonds, salt, and pepper.

INGREDIENTS

- 1 lb green beans, trimmed
- 1/4 cup sliced almonds
- 1 tbsp olive oil
- Salt and pepper to taste

Calories: 90, Protein: 3g, Carbs: 10g, Fat: 5g

Avocado Corn Salad

Prep Time: 10 minutes **Cook Time:** 0 minutes

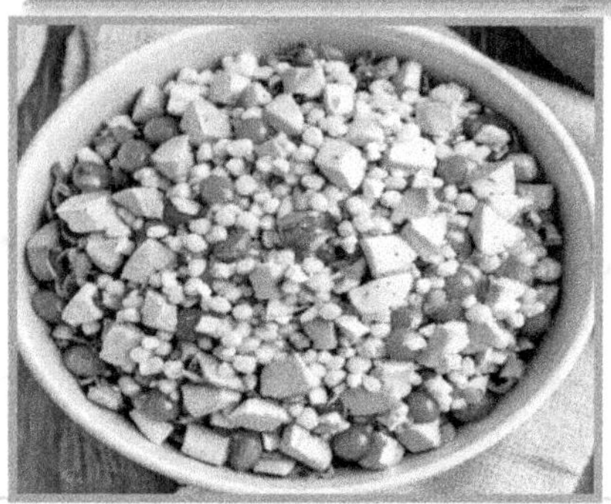

INSTRUCTIONS

1. In a bowl, combine avocados, corn, and red onion.
2. Drizzle with olive oil and lime juice.
3. Season with salt and pepper, and toss to combine.

INGREDIENTS

- 2 avocados, diced
- 1 cup corn kernels (fresh, frozen, or canned)
- 1/4 cup red onion, diced
- 1 tbsp olive oil
- 1 lime, juiced
- Salt and pepper to taste

Calories: 180, Protein: 2g, Carbs: 15g, Fat: 15g

Savory Additions

Garlic Mashed Cauliflower

Prep Time: 10 minutes **Cook Time:** 12 minutes

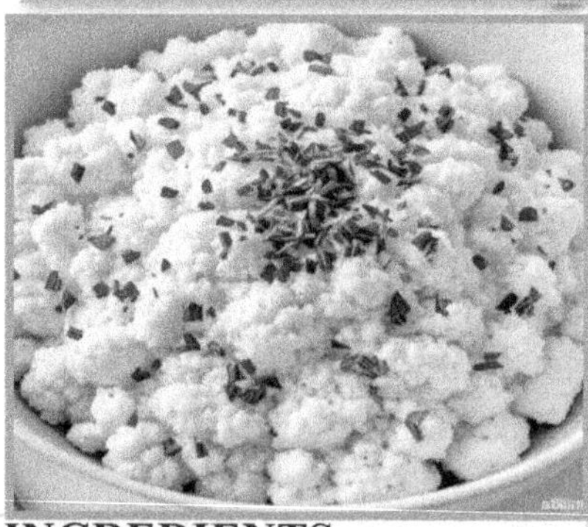

INSTRUCTIONS

1. Steam cauliflower until tender, about 10-12 minutes.
2. In a food processor, blend cauliflower, garlic, olive oil, salt, and pepper until smooth.

INGREDIENTS

- 1 head cauliflower, chopped
- 2 cloves garlic, minced
- 2 tbsp olive oil
- Salt and pepper to taste

Calories: 80, Protein: 2g, Carbs: 8g, Fat: 6g

Roasted Sweet Potatoes

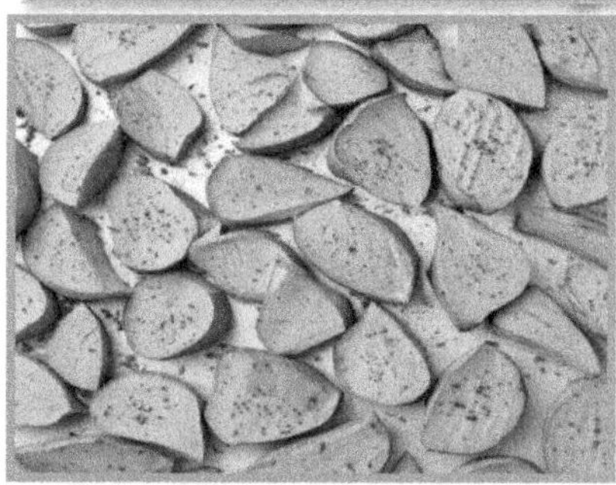

INSTRUCTIONS

1. Preheat oven to 425°F (220°C).
2. Toss sweet potatoes with olive oil, smoked paprika, salt, and pepper.
3. Spread on a baking sheet and roast for 25-30 minutes, until tender.

INGREDIENTS

- 2 sweet potatoes, diced
- 1 tbsp olive oil
- 1 tsp smoked paprika
- Salt and pepper to taste

Calories: 150, Protein: 2g, Carbs: 30g, Fat: 4g

Sautéed Spinach with Garlic

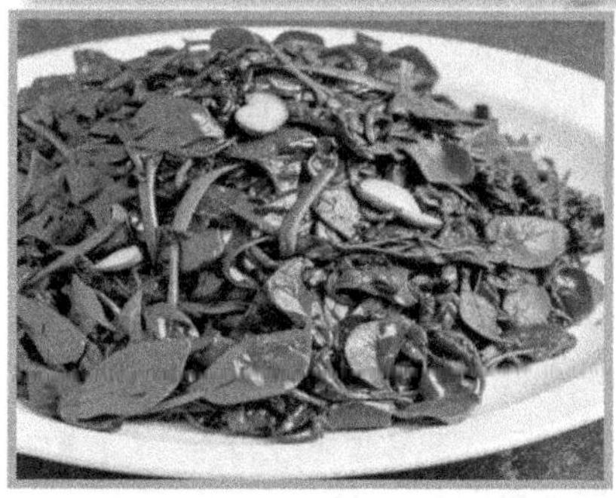

INSTRUCTIONS

1. In a large pan, heat olive oil over medium heat.
2. Add garlic and sauté for 1 minute.
3. Add spinach and cook until wilted, about 3-4 minutes.
4. Season with salt and pepper.

INGREDIENTS

- 1 lb spinach leaves
- 2 cloves garlic, minced
- 1 tbsp olive oil
- Salt and pepper to taste

Calories: 70, Protein: 3g, Carbs: 4g, Fat: 5g

Herb-Roasted Carrots

Prep Time: 10 minutes   **Cook Time:** 25 minutes

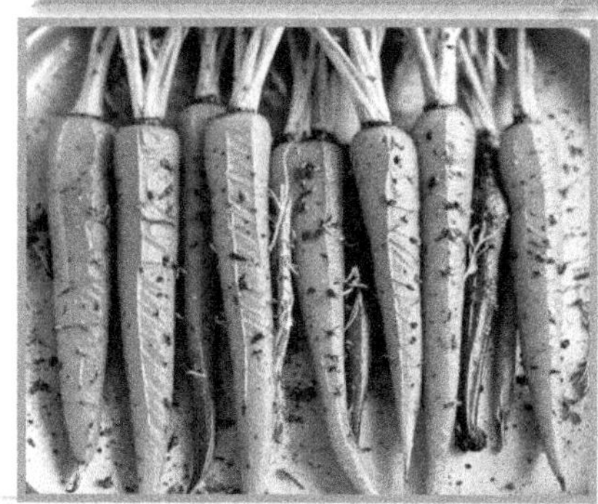

INSTRUCTIONS

1. Preheat oven to 400°F (200°C).
2. Toss carrots with olive oil, thyme, salt, and pepper.
3. Spread on a baking sheet and roast for 20-25 minutes, until tender.

INGREDIENTS

- 1 lb carrots, sliced
- 1 tbsp olive oil
- 1 tsp dried thyme
- Salt and pepper to taste

Calories: 100, Protein: 1g, Carbs: 15g, Fat: 4g

Brown Rice Pilaf

Prep Time: 10 minutes   **Cook Time:** 45 minutes

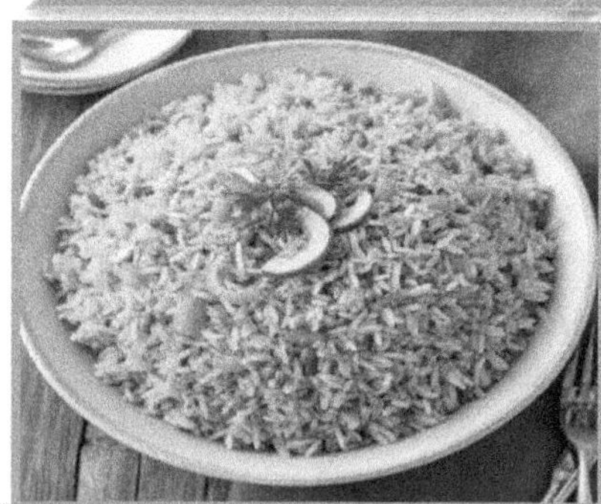

INSTRUCTIONS

1. In a pot, heat olive oil over medium heat.
2. Sauté onion and celery until soft, about 5 minutes.
3. Add brown rice and cook, stirring, for 2 minutes.
4. Add vegetable broth, bring to a boil, reduce heat, and simmer for 40-45

INGREDIENTS

- 1 cup brown rice
- 2 cups vegetable broth
- 1/4 cup diced onion
- 1/4 cup diced celery
- 1 tbsp olive oil
- Salt and pepper to taste

Calories: 180, Protein: 4g, Carbs: 35g, Fat: 4g

Chapter 6: Desserts

Snacking healthily may have a big influence on your energy levels and general health, according to American Heart Association studies. Snacks are an important part of the DASH diet because they help keep blood sugar levels in check and provide key nutrients in between meals. Simple but healthy snack options include almond butter on apple slices, hummus on vegetable sticks, and Greek yogurt with berries. These snacks are great for sating your appetite since they're high in fiber, protein, and good fats. They're also tasty.

You may maintain your nutritional objectives by including DASH-friendly snacks in your routine. Greek yogurt, for instance, is high in protein and probiotics, which help to maintain gut health and keep you feeling full. Hummus-topped veggie sticks make a crisp, filling snack that's rich in fiber and important vitamins. In the meanwhile, apple slices with almond butter provide a savory and sweet combo that is filling and healthy.

Snacking healthily also lessens the chance of overindulging during meals. Selecting foods high in nutrients can help you control your weight, strengthen your heart, and have steady energy levels all day. The DASH diet may be easily followed and made to seem like a fun part of your daily routine with the correct snacks.

Baked Cinnamon Apples

Prep Time: 10 minutes **Cook Time:** 25 minutes

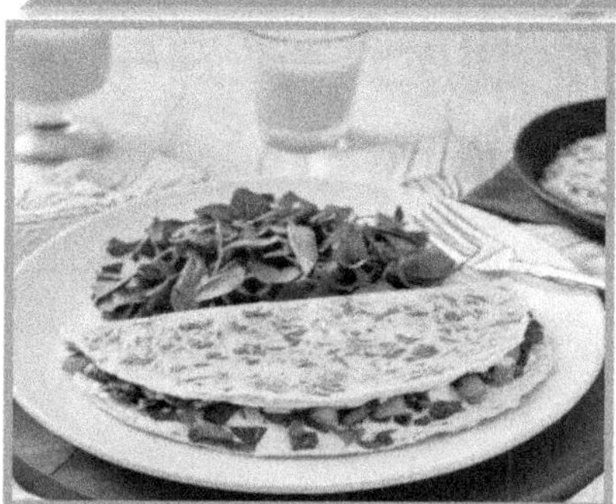

INGREDIENTS

- 4 large apples, cored and sliced
- 2 tbsp maple syrup
- 1 tsp cinnamon
- 1/4 cup chopped walnuts

INSTRUCTIONS

1. Preheat oven to 350°F (175°C).
2. Place apple slices in a baking dish.
3. Drizzle with maple syrup and sprinkle with cinnamon.
4. Top with chopped walnuts.
5. Bake for 20-25 minutes until apples are tender.

Calories: 150, Protein: 2g, Carbs: 32g, Fat: 4g

Greek Yogurt Parfait

Prep Time: 5 minutes **Cook Time:** 0 minutes

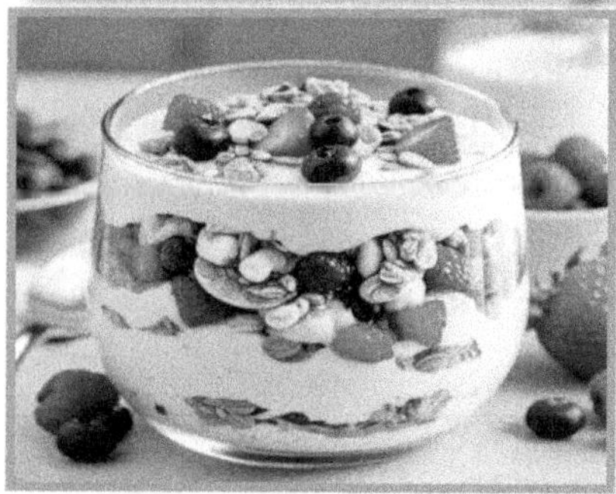

INGREDIENTS

- 1 cup Greek yogurt
- 1/2 cup mixed berries
- 1 tbsp honey
- 1/4 cup granola

INSTRUCTIONS

1. Layer Greek yogurt, mixed berries, and granola in a glass.
2. Drizzle with honey.

Calories: 250, Protein: 15g, Carbs: 35g, Fat: 8g

Dark Chocolate Almond Clusters

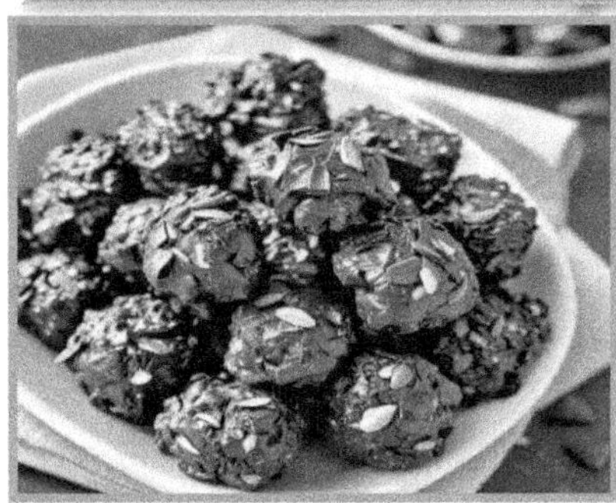

INGREDIENTS

INSTRUCTIONS

5. Melt dark chocolate chips in a microwave-safe bowl.
6. Stir in chopped almonds.
7. Drop spoonfuls onto a parchment-lined baking sheet.
8. Refrigerate until set.

- 1 cup dark chocolate chips
- 1/2 cup almonds, chopped

Calories: 120, Protein: 2g, Carbs: 15g, Fat: 8g

Chia Seed Pudding

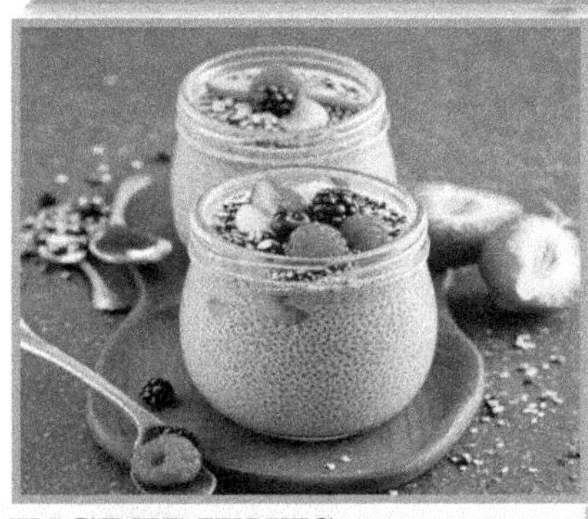

INGREDIENTS

INSTRUCTIONS

1. In a bowl, whisk almond milk, chia seeds, maple syrup, and vanilla extract.
2. Refrigerate for at least 4 hours or overnight, stirring occasionally.

- 1 cup almond milk
- 1/4 cup chia seeds
- 1 tbsp maple syrup
- 1/2 tsp vanilla extract

Calories: 200, Protein: 5g, Carbs: 20g, Fat: 10g

Banana Ice Cream

Prep Time: 5 minutes   **Cook Time:** 0 minutes

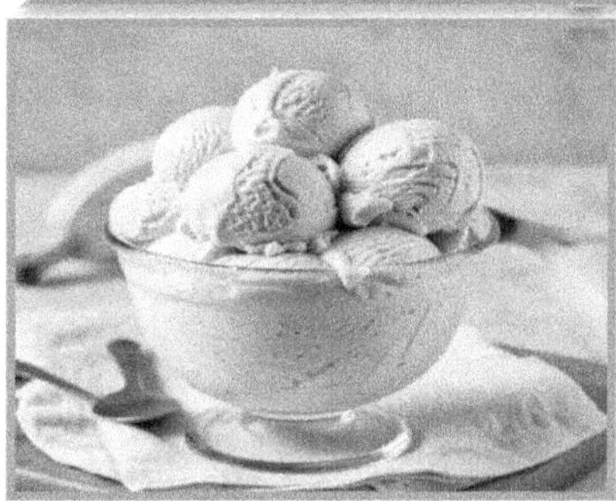

INSTRUCTIONS

1. Blend frozen banana slices and vanilla extract in a food processor until smooth.
2. Serve immediately or freeze for a firmer texture.

INGREDIENTS

- 2 ripe bananas, sliced and frozen
- 1 tsp vanilla extract

Calories: 100, Protein: 1g, Carbs: 25g, Fat: 0g

Fruity Delights

Berry Salad

Prep Time: 5 minutes   **Cook Time:** 0 minutes

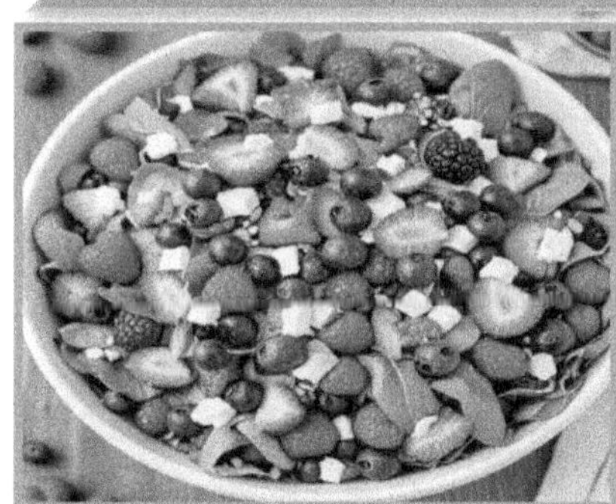

INSTRUCTIONS

1. Combine all berries in a large bowl.
2. Drizzle with lemon juice and honey.
3. Toss gently to combine.

INGREDIENTS

- 1 cup strawberries, sliced
- 1 cup blueberries
- 1 cup raspberries
- 1 tbsp lemon juice
- 1 tsp honey

Calories: 80, Protein: 1g, Carbs: 20g, Fat: 0g

Tropical Fruit Skewers

Prep Time: 10 minutes   **Cook Time:** 0 minutes

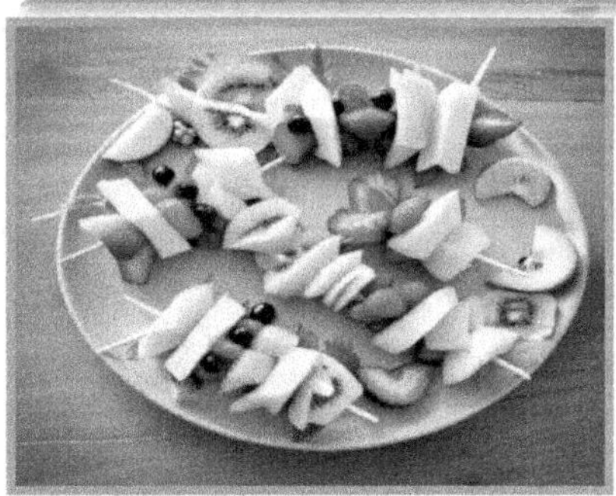

INSTRUCTIONS

1. Thread fruit onto skewers.
2. Serve immediately.

INGREDIENTS

- 1 mango, diced
- 1 pineapple, diced
- 2 kiwis, sliced
- 1 cup strawberries, hulled

Calories: 100, Protein: 1g, Carbs: 25g, Fat: 0g

Watermelon Feta Bites

Prep Time: 10 minutes   **Cook Time:** 0 minutes

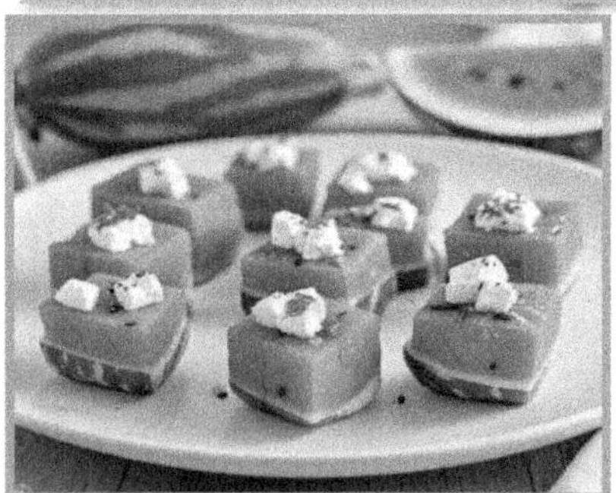

INSTRUCTIONS

1. Place a feta cheese crumble on each watermelon cube.
2. Garnish with a mint leaf.

INGREDIENTS

- 1 small watermelon, cut into cubes
- 1/2 cup feta cheese, crumbled
- Fresh mint leaves

Calories: 50, Protein: 2g, Carbs: 10g, Fat: 2g

Peach Yogurt Popsicles

Prep Time: 10 minutes **Cook Time:** 4hr freze

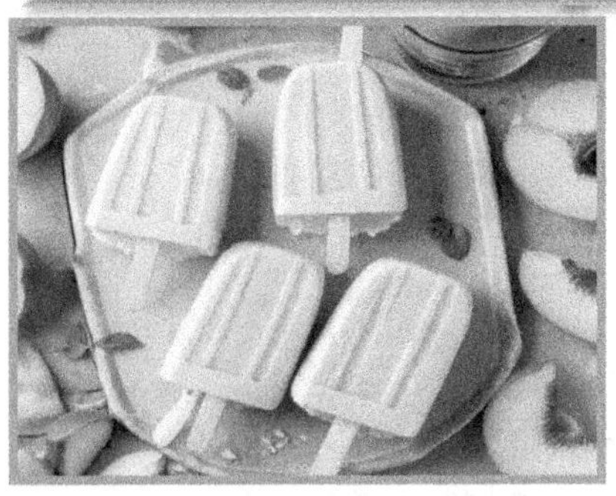

INSTRUCTIONS

1. Mix Greek yogurt, peach puree, and honey.
2. Pour mixture into popsicle molds.
3. Freeze for at least 4 hours.

INGREDIENTS

- 2 cups Greek yogurt
- 2 ripe peaches, pureed
- 1 tbsp honey

Calories: 80, Protein: 5g, Carbs: 15g, Fat: 1g

Orange Cream Smoothie

Prep Time: 10 minutes **Cook Time:** 0 minutes

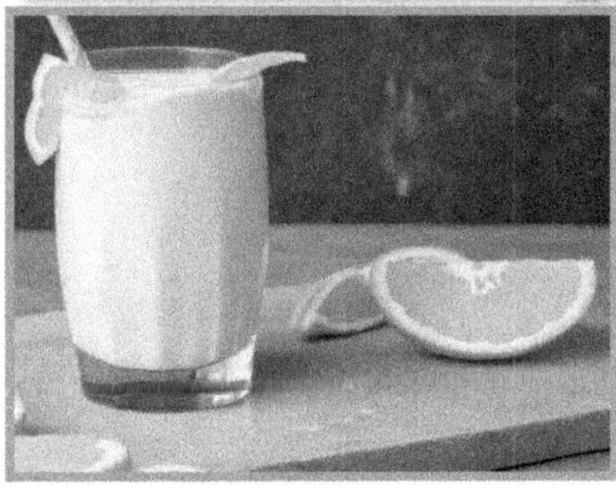

INSTRUCTIONS

1. Blend all ingredients until smooth.
2. Serve immediately.

INGREDIENTS

- 1 cup orange juice
- 1/2 cup Greek yogurt
- 1 banana
- 1 tsp vanilla extract

Calories: 150, Protein: 5g, Carbs: 30g, Fat: 1g

Lemon Sorbet

Prep Time: 10 minutes   **Cook Time:** 3hr freeze

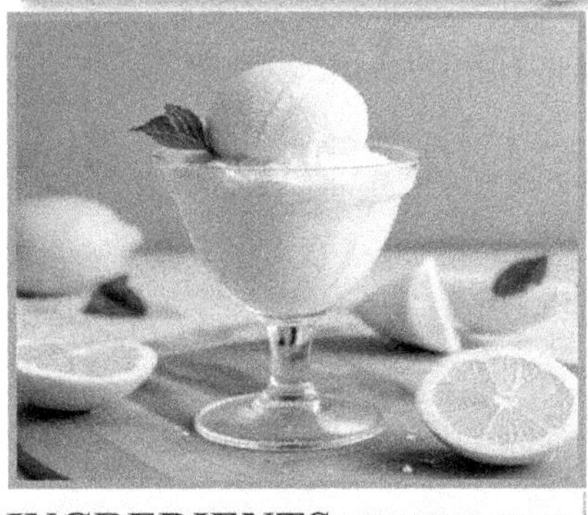

INSTRUCTIONS

1. Combine water and sugar in a saucepan and heat until sugar dissolves.
2. Stir in lemon juice and zest.
3. Pour into a shallow dish and freeze, stirring occasionally.

INGREDIENTS

- 1 cup water
- 1 cup sugar
- 1 cup lemon juice
- 1 tbsp lemon zest

Calories: 90, Protein: 0g, Carbs: 25g, Fat: 0g

Mango Lime Sorbet

Prep Time: 10 minutes   **Cook Time:** 3hr freeze

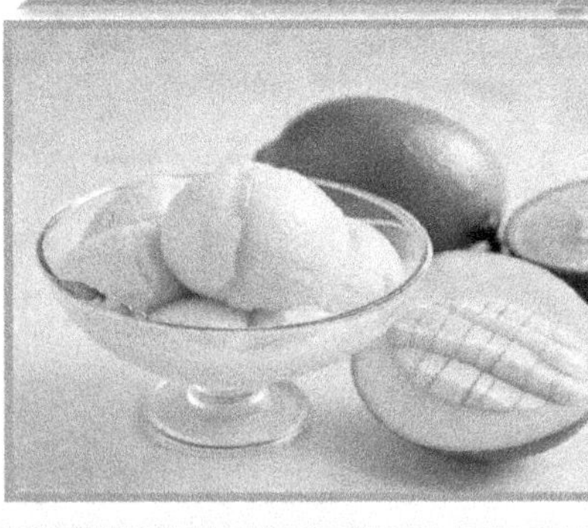

INSTRUCTIONS

1. Blend mangoes, lime juice, and honey until smooth.
2. Pour into a shallow dish and freeze, stirring occasionally.

INGREDIENTS

- 2 ripe mangoes, peeled and diced
- 1/4 cup lime juice
- 1/4 cup honey

Calories: 120, Protein: 1g, Carbs: 30g, Fat: 0g

Strawberry Basil Sorbet

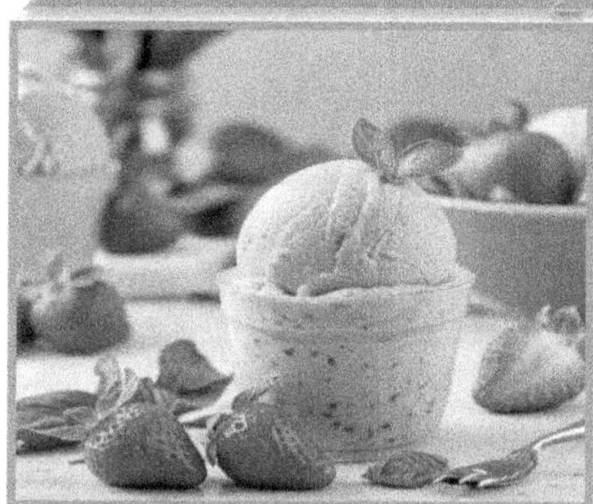

INSTRUCTIONS:

1. Blend strawberries, basil leaves, honey, and water until smooth.
2. Pour into a shallow dish and freeze, stirring occasionally.

INGREDIENTS

- 2 cups strawberries, hulled
- 1/4 cup basil leaves
- 1/4 cup honey
- 1/2 cup water

Calories: 80, Protein: 0g, Carbs: 20g, Fat: 0g

Cucumber Mint Granita

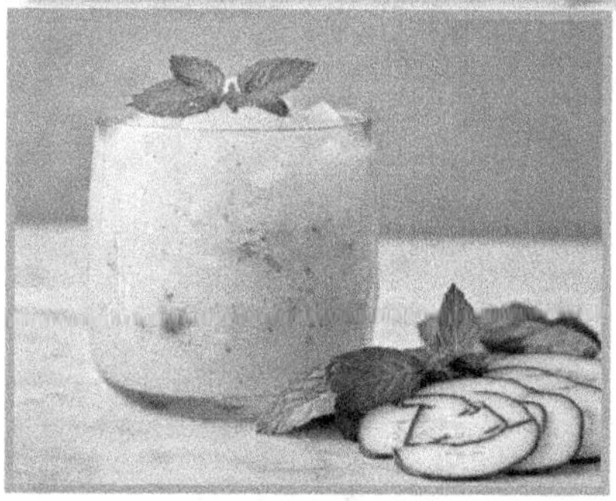

INSTRUCTIONS

1. Blend cucumbers, mint leaves, lime juice, and honey until smooth.
2. Pour into a shallow dish and freeze, stirring occasionally.

INGREDIENTS

- 2 cucumbers, peeled and diced
- 1/4 cup mint leaves
- 1/4 cup lime juice
- 1/4 cup honey

Calories: 60, Protein: 0g, Carbs: 15g, Fat: 0g

Pineapple Coconut Sorbet

Prep Time: 10 minutes   **Cook Time:** 3hrs freeze

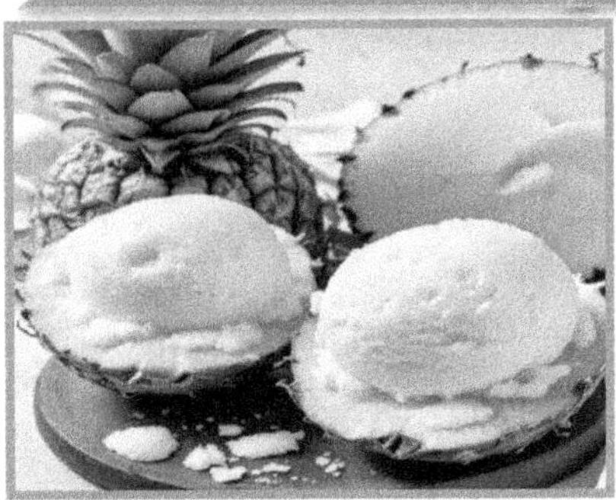

INSTRUCTIONS

1. Blend pineapple, coconut milk, and honey until smooth.
2. Pour into a shallow dish and freeze, stirring occasionally.

INGREDIENTS

- 1 pineapple, peeled and diced
- 1/2 cup coconut milk
- 1/4 cup honey

Calories: 100, Protein: 1g, Carbs: 25g, Fat: 1g

Indulgent Favorites

Chocolate Avocado Mousse

Prep Time: 10 minutes   **Cook Time:** 1hrs chill

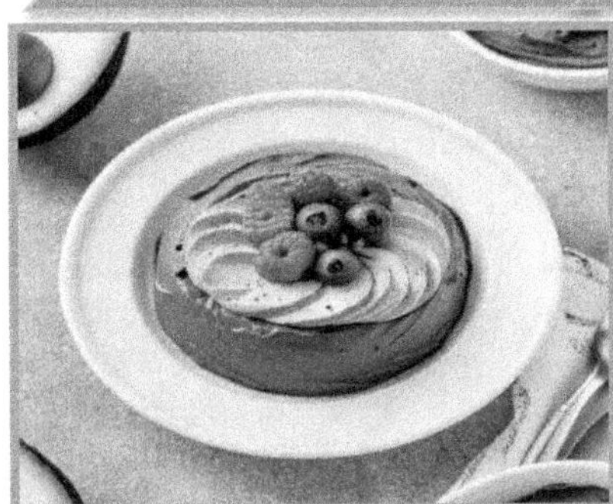

INSTRUCTIONS

1. Blend avocados, cocoa powder, honey, and vanilla extract until smooth.
2. Chill for 1 hour before serving.

INGREDIENTS

- 2 ripe avocados
- 1/4 cup cocoa powder
- 1/4 cup honey
- 1 tsp vanilla extract

Calories: 180, Protein: 2g, Carbs: 20g, Fat: 12g

Almond Flour Brownies

Prep Time: 10 minutes **Cook Time:** 25 minutes

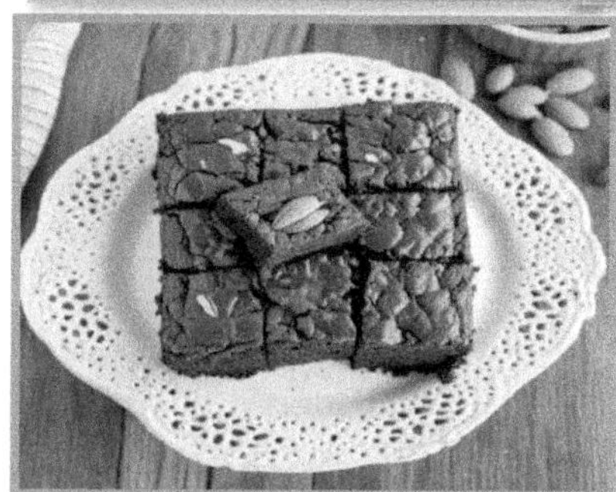

INSTRUCTIONS

1. Preheat oven to 350°F (175°C).
2. Mix all ingredients until well combined.
3. Pour into a greased baking dish.
4. Bake for 20-25 minutes.

INGREDIENTS

- 1 cup almond flour
- 1/2 cup cocoa powder
- 1/2 cup honey
- 2 eggs
- 1/4 cup coconut oil, melted
- 1 tsp vanilla extract

Calories: 150, Protein: 4g, Carbs: 20g, Fat: 8g

Raspberry Dark Chocolate Bark

Prep Time: 10 minutes **Cook Time:** 10 minutes

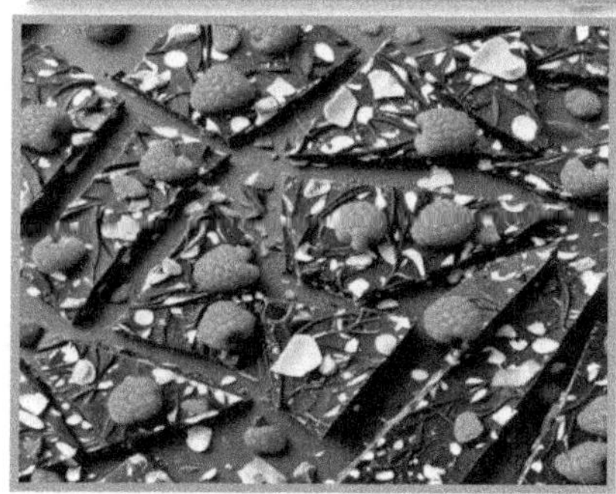

INSTRUCTIONS

1. Melt dark chocolate chips in a microwave-safe bowl.
2. Stir in freeze-dried raspberries.
3. Spread mixture onto a parchment-lined baking sheet.
4. Refrigerate until set.

INGREDIENTS

- 1 cup dark chocolate chips
- 1/2 cup freeze-dried raspberries

Calories: 120, Protein: 2g, Carbs: 15g, Fat: 8g

Coconut Macaroons

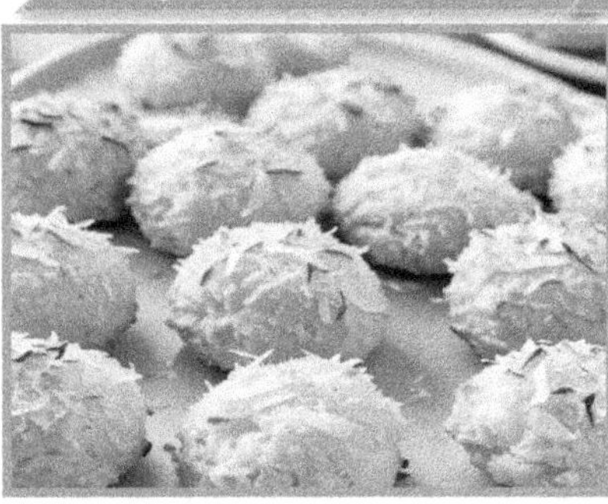

INSTRUCTIONS

1. Preheat oven to 325°F (165°C).
2. Mix all ingredients until well combined.
3. Drop spoonfuls onto a parchment-lined baking sheet.
4. Bake for 15-20 minutes.

INGREDIENTS

- 2 cups shredded coconut
- 1/2 cup honey
- 2 egg whites
- 1 tsp vanilla extract

Calories: 90, Protein: 1g, Carbs: 12g, Fat: 5g

Apple Crisp

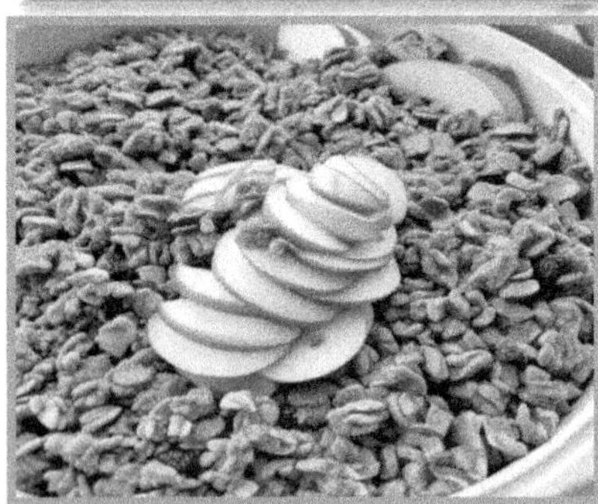

INSTRUCTIONS

1. Preheat oven to 350°F (175°C).
2. Place apple slices in a baking dish.
3. Mix oats, almond flour, honey, cinnamon, and coconut oil.
4. Sprinkle mixture over apples.
5. Bake for 30-35 minutes.

INGREDIENTS

- 4 apples, peeled and sliced
- 1/4 cup rolled oats
- 1/4 cup almond flour
- 1/4 cup honey
- 1 tsp cinnamon
- 1/4 cup coconut oil, melted

Calories: 180, Protein: 2g, Carbs: 30g, Fat: 8g

Chapter 7: 60-Day Meal Plan

The wise saying, ***"The journey of a thousand miles begins with one step,"*** which is sometimes credited to Lao Tzu, sums up exactly what it means to start a 60-day meal plan. Although the DASH diet may appear overwhelming at first, it is possible to guarantee a seamless transition to healthy eating habits by breaking it down into small stages. A well-defined plan will help ensure success throughout the first week of the travel, which is critical for establishing the tone for the remainder of the voyage.

You must get acquainted with the DASH diet's tenets and rules within the first week. The DASH diet limits foods rich in salt, added sugars, and saturated fats and emphasizes fruits, vegetables, whole grains, lean meats, and low-fat dairy. Recognizing these fundamental

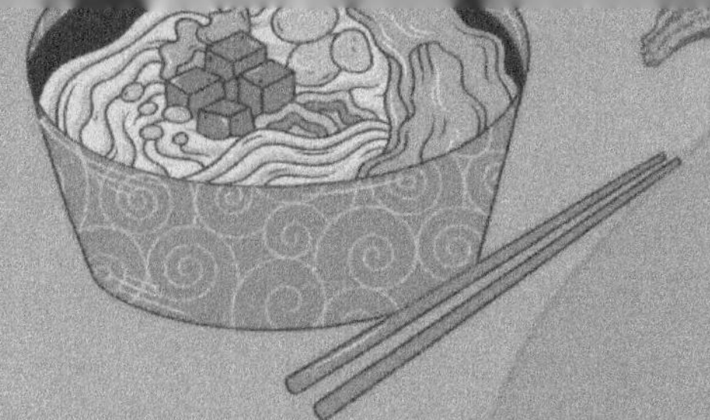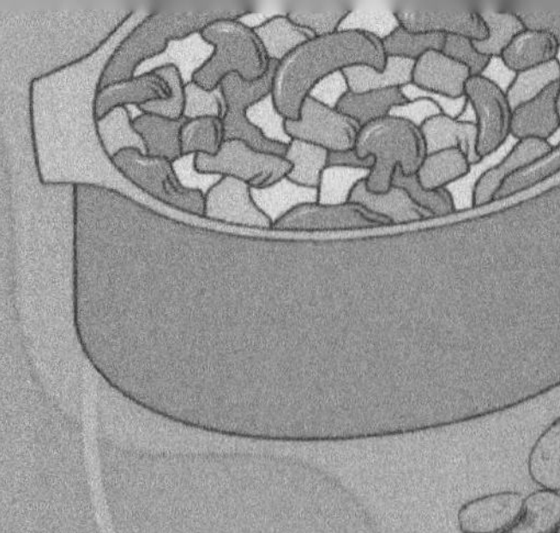

MEAL PLAN

DAY	BREAKFAST	LUNCH	DINNER
1	Berry Bliss Smoothie Bowl	Greek Salad	Lemon Herb Chicken and Vegetables
2	Classic Overnight Oats	Spinach and Strawberry Salad	Teriyaki Beef Stir-Fry
3	Blueberry Muffins	Chicken Caesar Salad	Garlic Shrimp and Asparagus
4	Veggie Omelet	Quinoa and Black Bean Salad	Italian Sausage and Peppers
5	Green Power Smoothie Bowl	Caprese Salad	Chicken Pot Pie
6	Apple Cinnamon Overnight Oats	Lentil Soup	Beef Stroganoff
7	Banana Bread	Chicken Noodle Soup	Shepherd's Pie

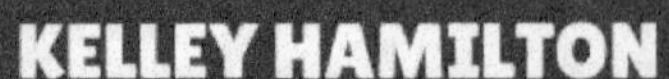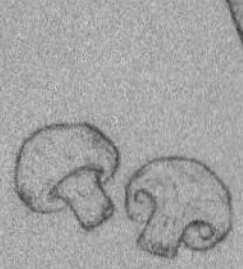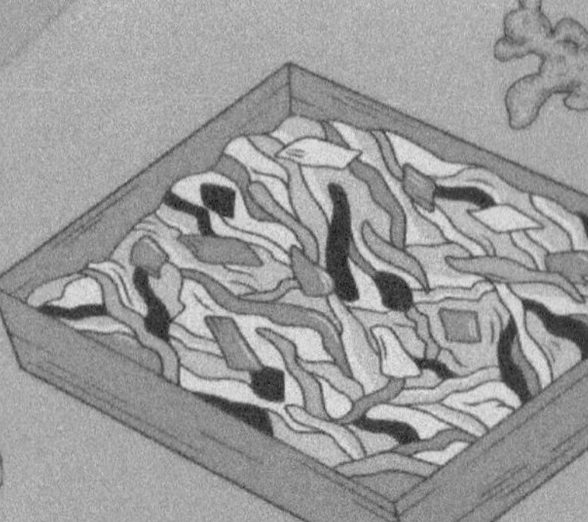

KELLEY HAMILTON

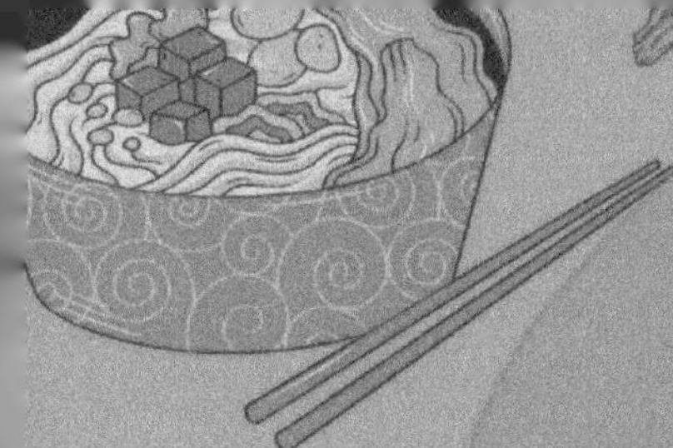
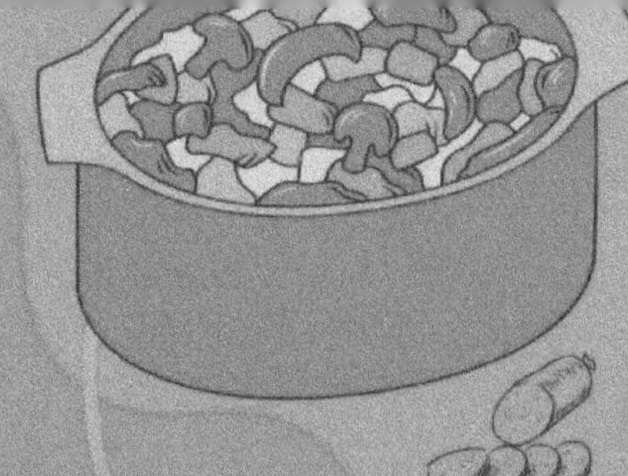

My 60-DAY
MEAL PLAN

DAY	BREAKFAST	LUNCH	DINNER
8	Cottage Cheese with Pineapple	Tomato Basil Soup	Meatloaf
9	Veggie Sticks with Hummus	Butternut Squash Soup	Lemon Herb Baked Salmon
10	Carrot Cake Muffins	Minestrone Soup	Garlic Shrimp Stir-Fry
11	Avocado Toast	Chicken Avocado Wrap	Grilled Tuna Steaks with Mango Salsa
12	Chocolate Peanut Butter Smoothie Bowl	Turkey and Hummus Wrap	Baked Cod with Tomatoes and Olives
13	Chocolate Almond Overnight Oats	Veggie Wrap	Shrimp and Avocado Salad
14	Zucchini Bread	Tuna Salad Wrap	Sweet Potato and Black Bean Chili

KELLEY HAMILTON

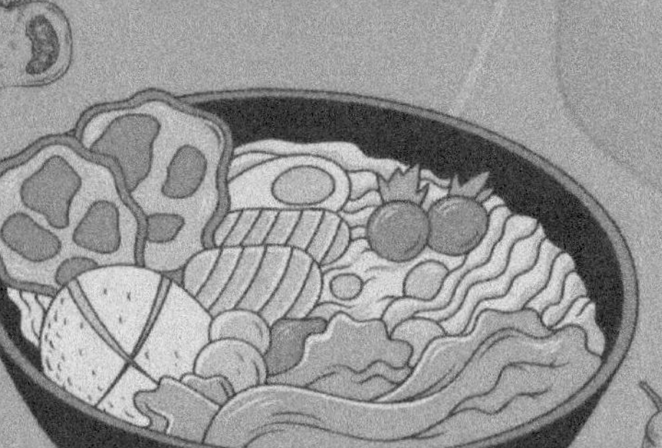
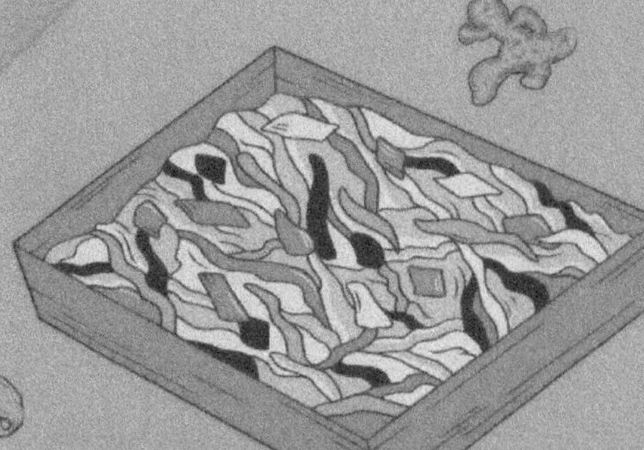

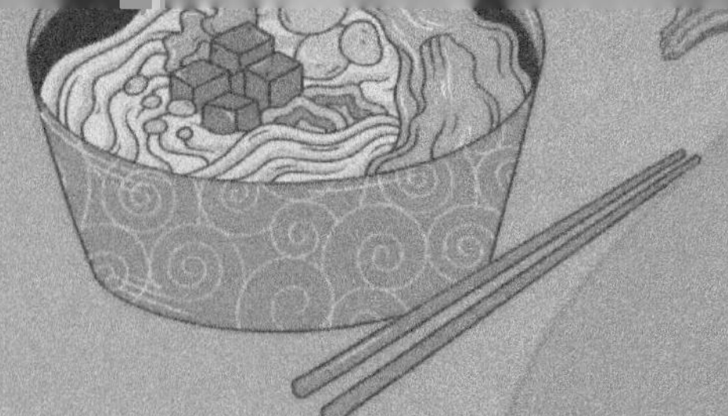
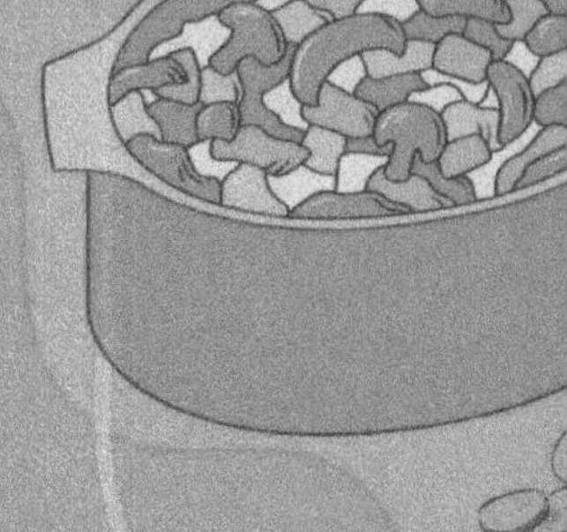

My 60-DAY
MEAL PLAN

DAY	BREAKFAST	LUNCH	DINNER
15	Acai Berry Smoothie Bowl	BBQ Chicken Wrap	Caprese Stuffed Portobello Mushrooms
16	Berry Vanilla Overnight Oats	Mediterranean Quinoa Bowl	Veggie Stir-Fry with Tofu
17	Apple Cinnamon Muffins	Teriyaki Chicken Rice Bowl	Spinach and Ricotta Stuffed Shells
18	Greek Yogurt Parfait	Southwest Black Bean Bowl	Mediterranean Chickpea Salad
19	Breakfast Burrito	Buddha Bowl	Lemon Herb Chicken and Vegetables
20	Steel-Cut Oats	Salmon and Brown Rice Bowl	Teriyaki Beef Stir-Fry
21	Berry Bliss Smoothie Bowl	Greek Salad	Garlic Shrimp and Asparagus

KELLEY HAMILTON

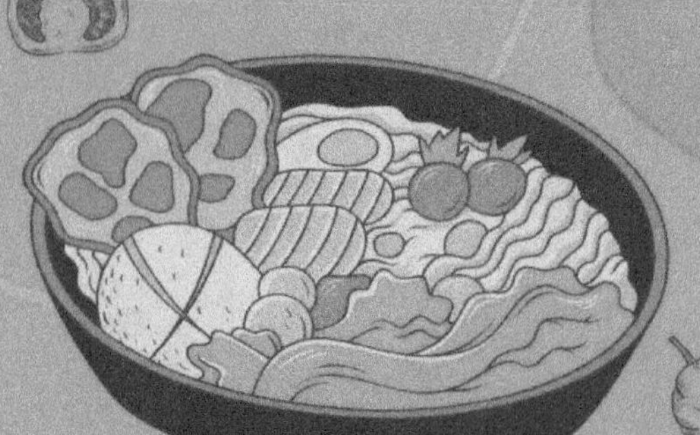
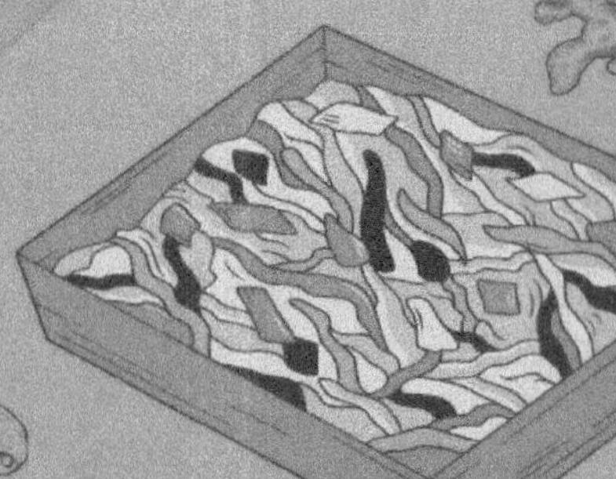

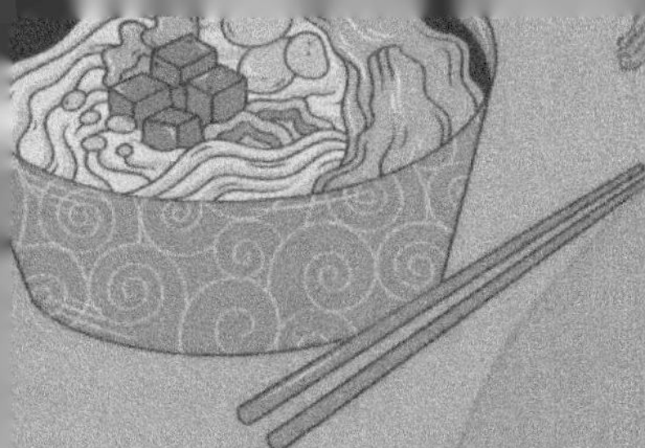
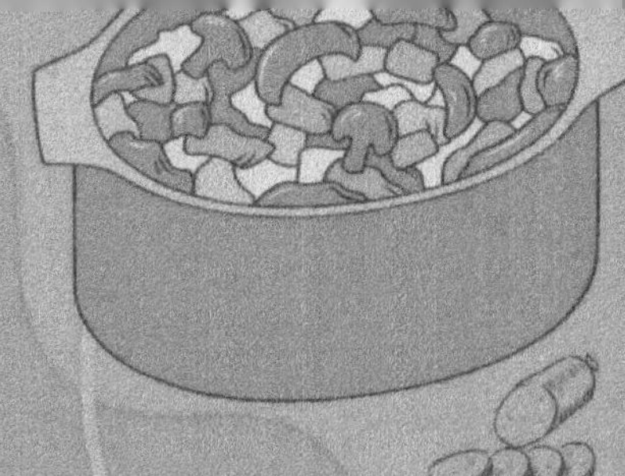

My 60-DAY
MEAL PLAN

DAY	BREAKFAST	LUNCH	DINNER
22	Classic Overnight Oats	Spinach and Strawberry Salad	Italian Sausage and Peppers
23	Blueberry Muffins	Chicken Caesar Salad	Chicken Pot Pie
24	Veggie Omelet	Quinoa and Black Bean Salad	Beef Stroganoff
25	Green Power Smoothie Bowl	Caprese Salad	Shepherd's Pie
26	Apple Cinnamon Overnight Oats	Lentil Soup	Meatloaf
27	Banana Bread	Chicken Noodle Soup	Lemon Herb Baked Salmon
28	Tropical Paradise Smoothie Bowl	Tomato Basil Soup	Garlic Shrimp Stir-Fry

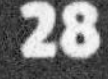
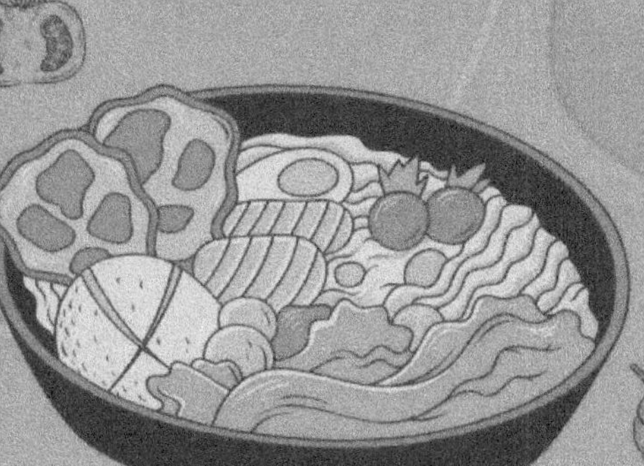

KELLEY HAMILTON

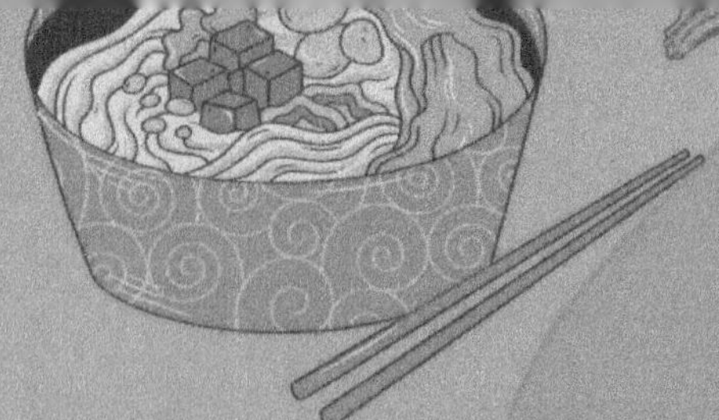
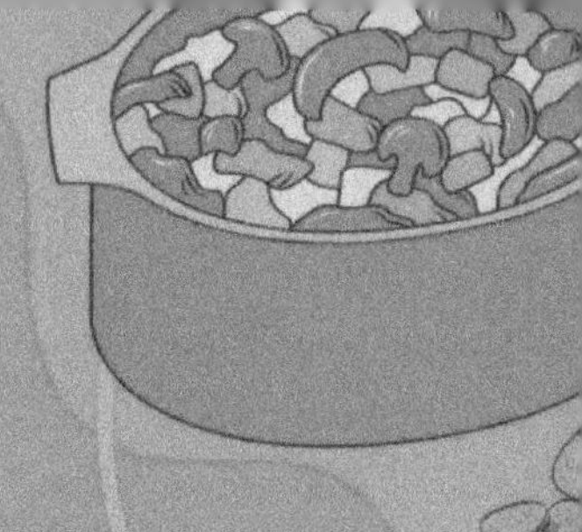

My 60-DAY
MEAL PLAN

DAY	BREAKFAST	LUNCH	DINNER
29	Peanut Butter Banana Overnight Oats	Butternut Squash Soup	Grilled Tuna Steaks with Mango Salsa
30	Carrot Cake Muffins	Minestrone Soup	Baked Cod with Tomatoes and Olives
31	Avocado Toast	Veggie Sticks with Hummus	Shrimp and Avocado Salad
32	Chocolate Peanut Butter Smoothie Bowl	Turkey and Hummus Wrap	Sweet Potato and Black Bean Chili
33	Chocolate Almond Overnight Oats	Veggie Wrap	Caprese Stuffed Portobello Mushrooms
34	Zucchini Bread	Tuna Salad Wrap	Veggie Stir-Fry with Tofu
35	Acai Berry Smoothie Bowl	BBQ Chicken Wrap	Spinach and Ricotta Stuffed Shells

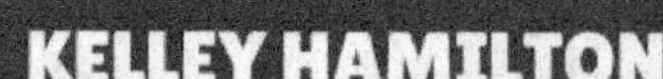
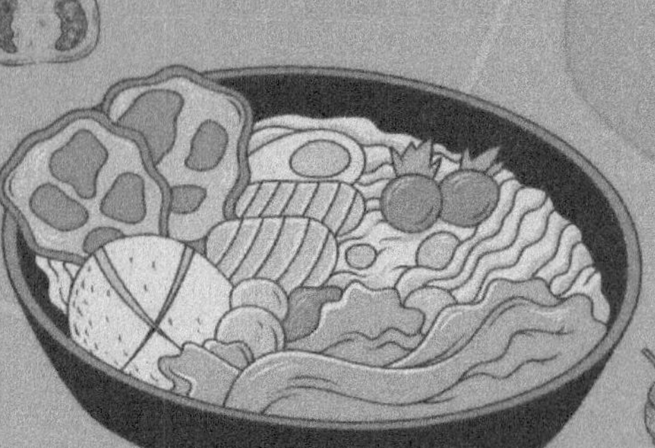
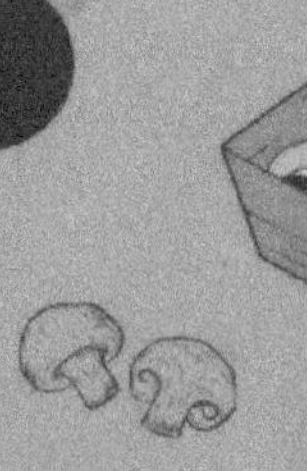

KELLEY HAMILTON

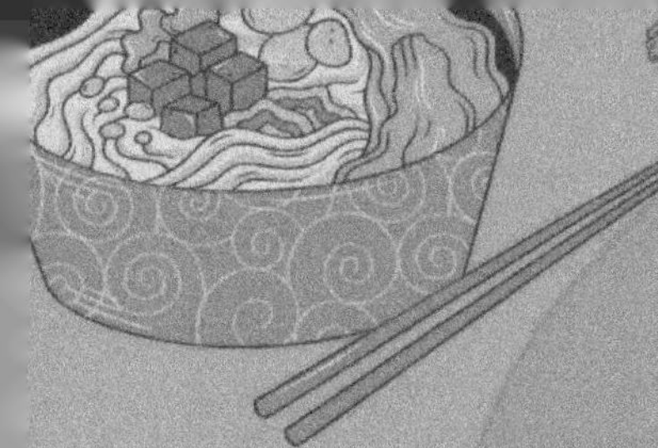
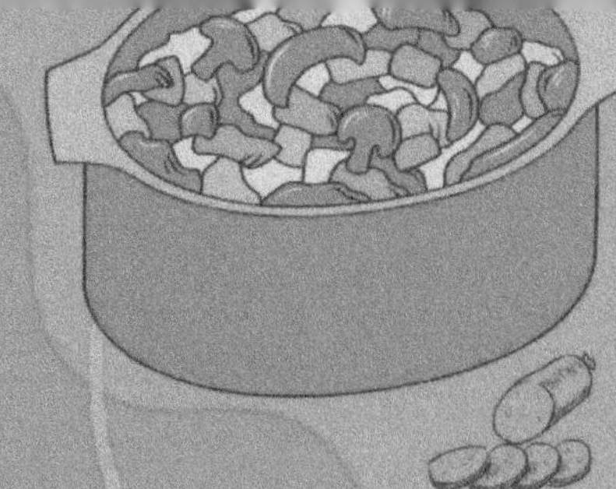

My 60-DAY
MEAL PLAN

DAY	BREAKFAST	LUNCH	DINNER
36	Berry Vanilla Overnight Oats	Mediterranean Quinoa Bowl	Mediterranean Chickpea Salad
37	Apple Cinnamon Muffins	Teriyaki Chicken Rice Bowl	Lemon Herb Chicken and Vegetables
38	Greek Yogurt Parfait	Southwest Black Bean Bowl	Teriyaki Beef Stir-Fry
39	Breakfast Burrito	Buddha Bowl	Garlic Shrimp and Asparagus
40	Steel-Cut Oats	Salmon and Brown Rice Bowl	Italian Sausage and Peppers
41	Berry Bliss Smoothie Bowl	Greek Salad	Chicken Pot Pie
42	Classic Overnight Oats	Spinach and Strawberry Salad	Beef Stroganoff

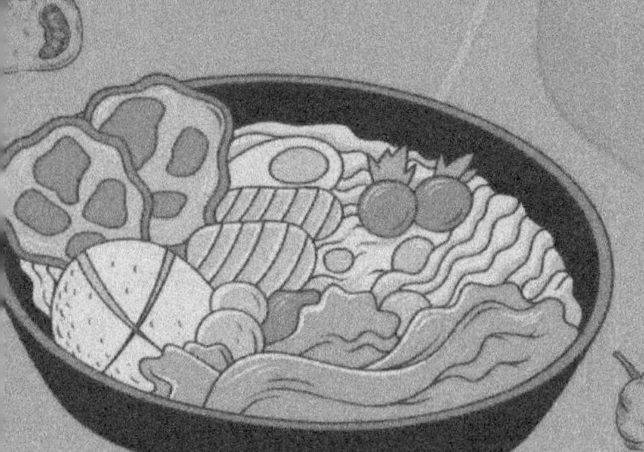

KELLEY HAMILTON

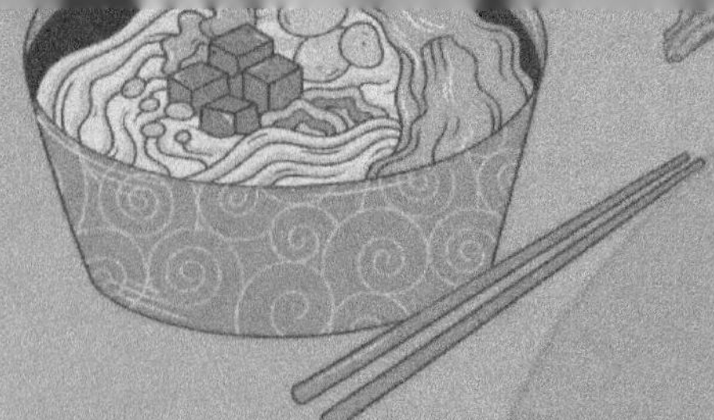
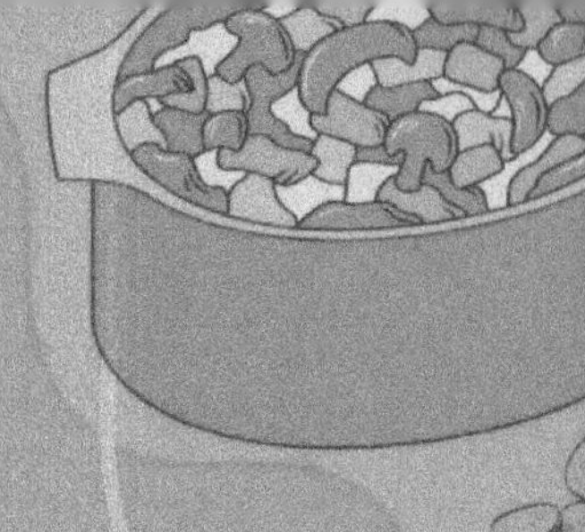

My 60-DAY
MEAL PLAN

DAY	BREAKFAST	LUNCH	DINNER
43	Blueberry Muffins	Chicken Caesar Salad	Shepherd's Pie
44	Veggie Omelet	Quinoa and Black Bean Salad	Meatloaf
45	Green Power Smoothie Bowl	Caprese Salad	Lemon Herb Baked Salmon
46	Apple Cinnamon Overnight Oats	Lentil Soup	Garlic Shrimp Stir-Fry
47	Banana Bread	Chicken Noodle Soup	Grilled Tuna Steaks with Mango Salsa
48	Tropical Paradise Smoothie Bowl	Tomato Basil Soup	Baked Cod with Tomatoes and Olives
49	Peanut Butter Banana Overnight Oats	Butternut Squash Soup	Shrimp and Avocado Salad

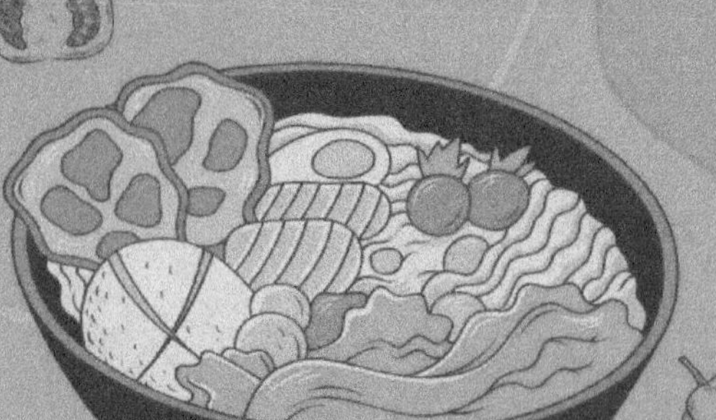
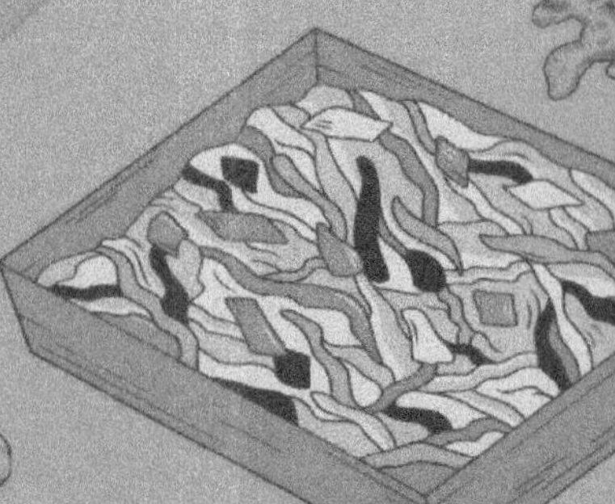

KELLEY HAMILTON

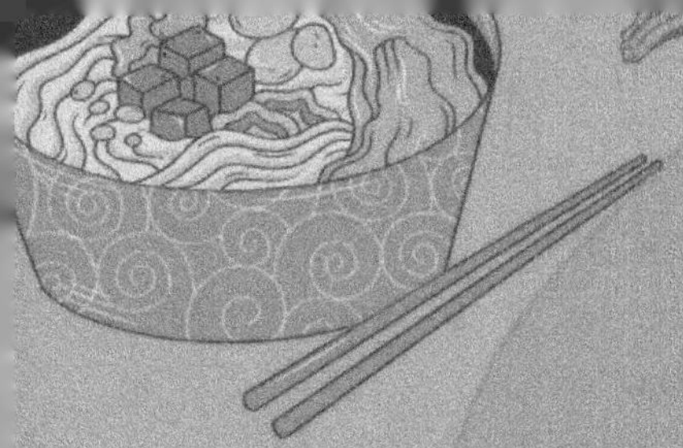
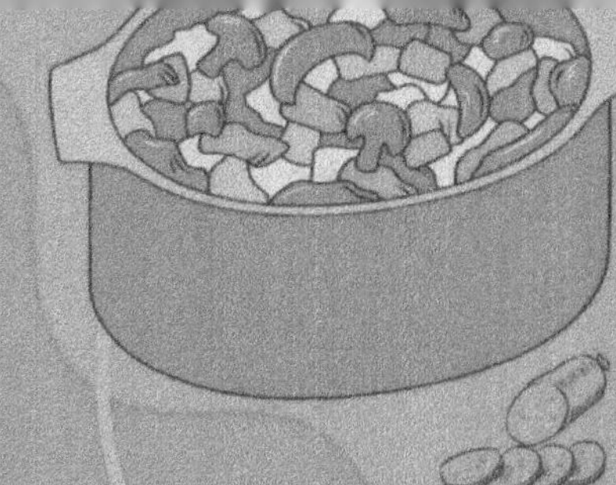

My 60-DAY
MEAL PLAN

DAY	BREAKFAST	LUNCH	DINNER
50	Carrot Cake Muffins	Minestrone Soup	Sweet Potato and Black Bean Chili
51	Avocado Toast	Chicken Avocado Wrap	Caprese Stuffed Portobello Mushrooms
52	Chocolate Peanut Butter Smoothie Bowl	Turkey and Hummus Wrap	Veggie Stir-Fry with Tofu
53	Chocolate Almond Overnight Oats	Veggie Wrap	Spinach and Ricotta Stuffed Shells
54	Zucchini Bread	Tuna Salad Wrap	Mediterranean Chickpea Salad
55	Acai Berry Smoothie Bowl	BBQ Chicken Wrap	Lemon Herb Chicken and Vegetables
56	Berry Vanilla Overnight Oats	Mediterranean Quinoa Bowl	Teriyaki Beef Stir-Fry

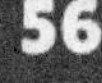
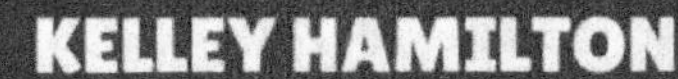
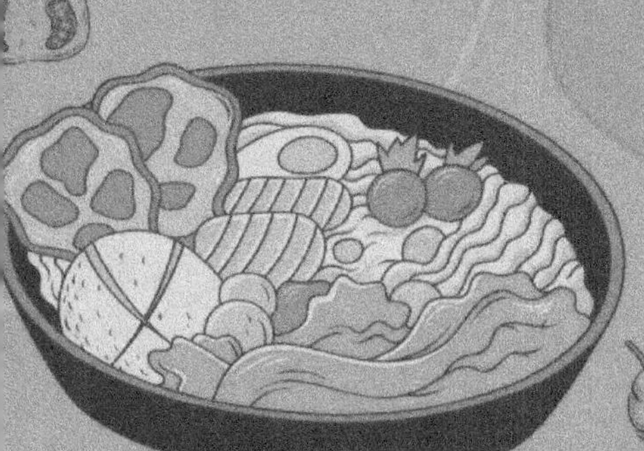

KELLEY HAMILTON

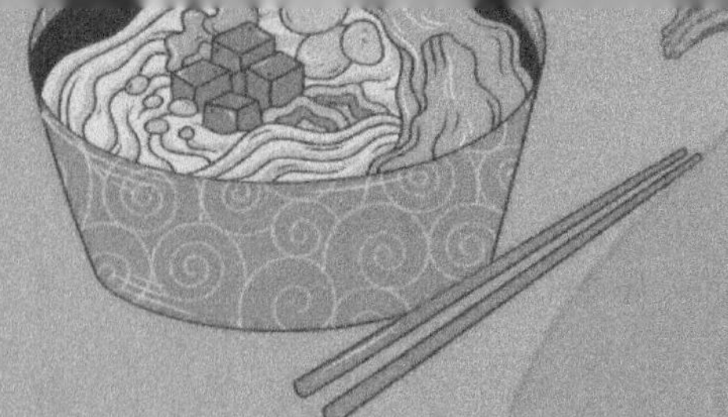
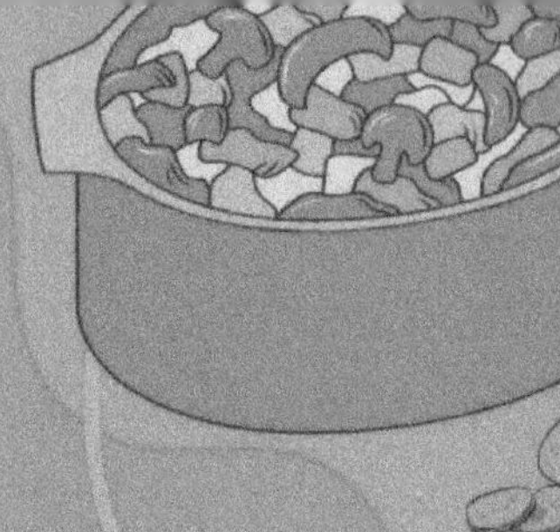

My 60-DAY
MEAL PLAN

DAY	BREAKFAST	LUNCH	DINNER
57	Apple Cinnamon Muffins	Teriyaki Chicken Rice Bowl	Garlic Shrimp and Asparagus
58	Greek Yogurt Parfait	Southwest Black Bean Bowl	Italian Sausage and Peppers
59	Breakfast Burrito	Buddha Bowl	Chicken Pot Pie
60	Steel-Cut Oats	Salmon and Brown Rice Bowl	Beef Stroganoff

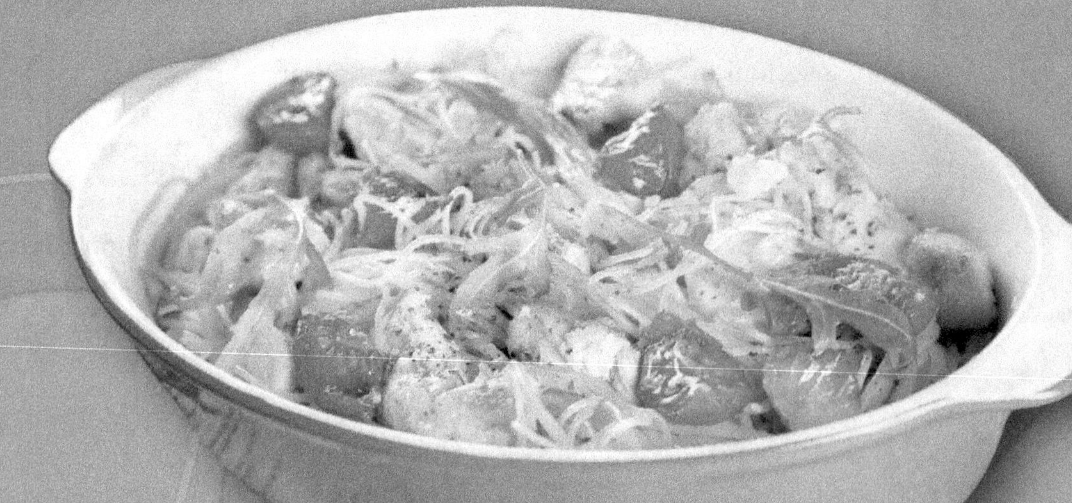

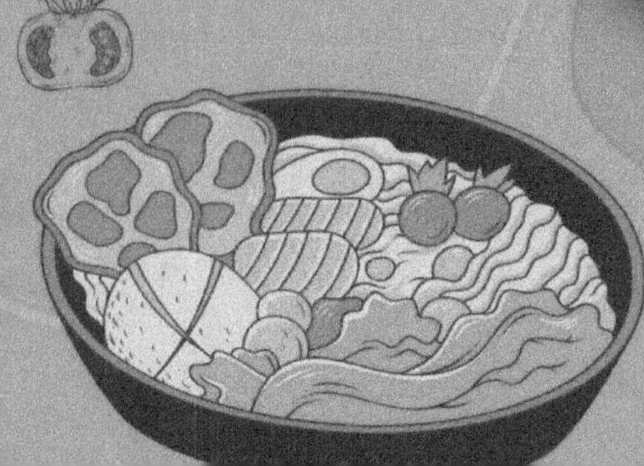

KELLEY HAMILTON

Chapter 8

Expert Tips and Resources

Grocery Shopping Tips for the DASH Diet

Benjamin Franklin famously said, "An investment in knowledge pays the best interest." This adage is especially valid for food shopping related to the DASH diet. Gaining the appropriate information may have a big impact on the quality of your meals and, in turn, your overall health. Dietary Approaches to Stop Hypertension, or DASH diet, emphasizes heart-healthy eating habits that may help decrease blood pressure. To make sure you're obtaining the healthiest alternatives, grocery shopping for this diet requires careful planning, label reading, and ingredient selection.

Making a thoughtful list is the first step in starting your food shopping trip. A range of fruits, vegetables, whole grains, lean meats, and low-fat dairy products should be on this list. The DASH diet is based on these food categories, which are low in sodium and saturated fat and high in fiber, protein, potassium, calcium, and magnesium. Making a plan and preparing your meals and snacks in advance can help you stay on track and prevent impulsive purchases that may not be by the DASH diet recommendations.

One of the most important skills to master for a successful DASH diet grocery shopping is reading labels. Look at the serving size and the quantity of servings per container first. This will assist you in realizing how much you're eating since the nutritional data is based on a single serving size. To control your total calorie consumption, next, check the calories per serving.

Keep a close eye on the salt amount specified on the label. According to the DASH diet, consuming no more than 2,300 milligrams of salt daily—ideally, only 1,500 milligrams for even more blood pressure reduction. Select goods with the labels "no added salt," "low sodium," or "reduced sodium." When feasible, choose fresh or frozen meals instead of processed and packaged ones since they often include high amounts of salt, such as canned vegetables, soups, and deli meats.

Dietary fiber is another important component to keep an eye on. The DASH diet requires a lot of foods rich in fiber, such as fruits, vegetables, and whole grains. Choose goods that provide three grams or more of fiber per serving. Whole grain alternatives such as oats, brown rice, quinoa, and whole wheat pasta are great options. Look for "whole grain" or "whole wheat" as the first component stated when choosing bread or cereal.

Selecting lean proteins is yet another crucial DASH diet component. Fish, lentils, legumes, almonds, and skinless chicken are all great sources of lean protein. Pick beef pieces marked "loin" or "round," since they are often lower in fat. Furthermore, include a few times a week in your diet foods high in omega-3 fatty acids, such as salmon, mackerel, and sardines.

Dairy products must be fat-free or low-fat to comply with the DASH diet guidelines. Select reduced-fat cheese, yogurt, and skim milk. Without the additional saturated fat included in full-fat dairy products, these choices provide the required amounts of calcium and vitamin D.

The DASH diet's mainstays are fruits and vegetables because of their high nutritional density and low-calorie content. Pick a diverse assortment of produce when you go grocery shopping to make sure you're receiving a mix of vitamins, minerals, and antioxidants. Fruits and vegetables may be included in a healthy diet either fresh, frozen, or canned; if you choose to can them, be sure there are no added sugars or salt.

The DASH diet includes healthy fats as well, but it's crucial to choose the appropriate kinds and consume them in moderation. Canola, avocado, and olive oils are good sources of polyunsaturated and monounsaturated fatty acids. Nuts and seeds that include healthy fats, including flaxseeds, walnuts, and almonds, may be added to meals and snacks to boost their nutritional value.

Since fresh vegetables, meats, and dairy goods are usually found along the perimeter of the grocery store, shopping there is a useful technique. The middle aisles are often where you'll find processed and packaged goods, which are frequently higher in added sugars and salt. Don't completely disregard these aisles, either, since they do include vital products like beans and nutritious grains. Rather, thoroughly study labels and choose the healthiest alternatives available.

Following the DASH diet requires you to be a knowledgeable and conscientious consumer. Making nutrient-dense food choices, organizing your shopping excursions, and reading labels can help you make better decisions that will support your overall health and blood pressure control. Recall that devoting time and energy to comprehending what enters your body is an investment in your lifespan and overall health.

Time-Saving Meal Prep Techniques

The famous quote from Peter Drucker, "Time is the scarcest resource and unless it is managed nothing else can be managed," emphasizes how crucial effective time management is, particularly when it comes to preparing meals. Using time-saving meal preparation strategies may help the cooking process become more sustainable and doable while adhering to the DASH diet guidelines.

The method of batch cooking is among the best. Set aside several hours per week to cook more of the basic ingredients—like grains, meats, and vegetables—in bigger amounts. Grain grains such as brown rice or quinoa may be portioned and refrigerated for easy weekday meals. In a similar vein, split up tofu or roasted or grilled chicken breasts into containers for quick additions to salads, wraps, or grain bowls.

Using instant pots or slow cookers is another time-saving tip. These culinary tools are ideal for making soups, stews, and braised foods since they enable hands-off cooking. All you have to do is add your ingredients in the morning or early afternoon, set a timer, and return to a healthy dinner that is prepared for serving.

Preparing fruits and vegetables in advance may cut down on prep time considerably. Purchase a high-quality mandolin slicer or vegetable chopper to rapidly chop or slice veggies for stir-fries, salads, or snacks. To ensure easy access throughout the week, store pre-cut veggies in the refrigerator in airtight containers or zipper bags.

Another clever time-saver is to use frozen fruits and vegetables. Produce that is frozen is often pre-washed, and pre-cut, and still has some nutritional value. For extra convenience without sacrificing nutrition, try adding frozen mixed veggies to soups, casseroles, or stir-fries, or use frozen berries in smoothies.

It's essential to plan and arrange your meal prep ahead of time. Based on the DASH diet guidelines, make a weekly food plan that includes breakfast, lunch, supper, and snacks. This makes grocery shopping easier and guarantees you have all the components on hand. Meal prep that is portioned ahead of time into individual serving sizes or mason jars encourages portion management, which makes it simpler to maintain your nutritional objectives.

Finally, embrace quick and flexible recipes that call for little preparation time and supplies. Choose sheet pan dinners, salads that can be dressed up or down with various components, or one-pot meals. This method shortens the time spent cooking and cleaning up afterward, making meal preparation less stressful and more pleasurable.

Through the use of these efficient meal preparation methods, you may effectively integrate the DASH diet's tenets into your everyday schedule. Having wholesome meals on hand is guaranteed by efficient time management in the kitchen, which promotes your general health and well-being over time.

Portion Control and Mindful Eating

The Centers for Disease Management and Prevention (CDC) stresses that "good nutrition is an important part of leading a healthy lifestyle," emphasizing the importance of portion management and mindful eating in preserving general well-being. These techniques are essential to the DASH diet because they encourage better eating habits as well as efficient weight and blood pressure control.

Understanding and controlling how much food you eat at each meal and snack is known as portion control. Even when eating wholesome meals in excess, overeating may result in a calorie surplus and weight gain. You may more effectively monitor your calorie consumption and achieve weight management objectives by regulating portion sizes. Using smaller plates and bowls, measuring quantities using cups or scales, and splitting meals into proper serving sizes before eating are all useful strategies for portion management.

Beyond just watching your portion sizes, mindful eating emphasizes the whole quality of your mealtime experience. It entails eating mindfully, appreciating every meal, and paying attention to signals of hunger and fullness. Eating mindfully lowers the risk of overindulging and improves digestion while fostering a positive connection with food. To eat mindfully, turn off electronics like televisions and cellphones during meals, chew food well, and take pauses in between mouthfuls to gauge your degree of hunger.

Adherence to the DASH diet guidelines is supported when you include these behaviors in your routine. You may improve digestion, maintain a healthy weight, and increase the nutritional value of your meals by paying closer attention to portion sizes and eating habits. In the end, developing mindful eating and portion restriction as lifestyle habits promotes long-term health and well-being, which is in perfect harmony with the DASH diet's objectives for heart health and general vigor.

Staying Motivated and Overcoming Challenges

When starting a DASH diet, Winston Churchill's quote, "Success is not final, failure is not fatal: It is the courage to continue that counts," strikes a deep chord. Any new diet plan might have difficulties when starting, but they can be avoided to attain long-term health advantages if you are determined and prepared ahead of time.

Decreasing salt consumption is a frequent adjustment problem for those beginning the DASH diet. Today's diets are mostly made up of packaged and processed foods, which often have excessive salt content. It takes careful reading of labels and selection of lower-sodium substitutes when making the switch to fresh, natural foods. Try experimenting with different herbs and spices for flavor and gradually modify your taste preferences to overcome this difficulty. You should also progressively limit your consumption of salt over time.

Continuing to be consistent and motivated is another challenge. Maintaining the DASH diet takes dedication and persistence, just like any other lifestyle adjustment. Encouraging people to stay motivated may be achieved by setting reasonable objectives, such as adding one new DASH-friendly meal each week or gradually increasing fruit and vegetable portions. To remain motivated and responsible, acknowledge your little victories along the road and ask for help from loved ones, friends, or online networks.

It might also be intimidating to plan and prepare meals at first. Make time every week to plan meals, make shopping lists, and prepare items ahead of time to overcome this issue. For inspiration and direction, make use of resources like recipe books, meal-planning apps, and internet forums. To ensure that there are nutritious alternatives accessible on hectic days, batch preparing and portioning meals into containers may save time.

The last difficulty with following the DASH diet is managing social settings and eating out. To be ready, go over the menus in advance of the restaurant, ask to have meals modified to include more vegetables or less salt, and speak up when expressing dietary wishes. Provide healthy snack alternatives at social events by bringing DASH-friendly foods.

Never forget that adopting a DASH diet is a journey rather than a sprint. Remember the advantages for your health, such as lower blood pressure and heart health, and acknowledge and appreciate each accomplishment. You may effectively implement the DASH diet into your lifestyle and get the long-term benefits of a well-balanced and nutrient-rich diet by accepting obstacles as chances for personal development and education.

Chapter 9
Nutritional Information and Glossary

Understanding Nutritional Labels

The significance of knowing what our bodies are nourished with. Learning to read and understand nutritional labels is essential when starting the DASH diet to make well-informed food choices that promote heart health and general well-being.

Essential details regarding the nutrients included in packaged foods are provided via nutritional labels. Their purpose is to assist customers in making well-informed choices about their food consumption. When reading nutrition labels, keep an eye out for the following important details:

- ❖ **Serving Size:** The quantity of food needed to determine the remaining nutritional values is determined by this information, which is the first item on the label. To determine your precise nutritional consumption, pay attention to the serving size.
- ❖ **Calories:** The amount of energy in a food item is indicated by the number of calories per serving. It's important to keep an eye on your calorie consumption for both general health and weight control.
- ❖ **Find out about the macronutrients**—fats, proteins, and carbs. While reducing saturated and trans fats, the DASH diet promotes the intake of complex carbs, lean proteins, and healthy fats.
- ❖ **Sodium:** Those on the DASH diet must pay close attention to the amount of sodium they consume since too much salt may raise blood pressure. Choose items that are labeled as having less salt or low sodium.
- ❖ **Dietary fiber** may help decrease cholesterol levels and is necessary for the functioning of the digestive system. To promote heart health, choose high-fiber meals including fruits, vegetables, and whole grains.
- ❖ **Added Sugars:** Take caution while consuming added sugars as they may increase caloric intake without offering any nutritional advantages. Choose meals with as little added sugar as possible and concentrate on naturally sweet foods like fruits.
- ❖ **Minerals and vitamins:** Vitamin and mineral content in food may be included on nutritional labels. Seek for meals high in minerals like magnesium, calcium, and potassium, since they are crucial for preserving blood pressure within normal limits.

Comprehending and analyzing nutritional labels enables people to make knowledgeable choices consistent with the DASH diet's tenets. You may successfully promote heart health and general well-being by choosing foods low in salt, saturated fats, and added sugars and high in important nutrients. Recall that you are better able to fuel your body and reach your health objectives the more knowledgeable you are about the ingredients in your diet.

Glossary of Common Terms and Ingredients

Sir Francis Bacon is credited with saying, "Knowledge is power," and this is particularly true while traversing the fields of nutrition and culinary arts. A dictionary of common terminology and ingredients is a useful tool for novices starting the DASH diet to improve comprehension and confidence while preparing meals.

Key terminology and ingredients that are regularly found in the cookbook and the DASH diet recommendations are defined and explained in the glossary. How it may help readers is as follows:

- ❖ **Definitions:** The glossary dispels myths about words that are often used in dietary recommendations and recipes. For example, concise definitions of phrases like "whole grains," "lean proteins," and "low-fat dairy" assist readers in understanding the significance of these foods in the DASH diet.
- ❖ The DASH diet recommends several items, such as "quinoa," "chia seeds," and "nutritional yeast." This section provides information on these substances. Readers will be able to make educated decisions based on their dietary requirements and preferences if each post includes culinary advice, nutritional advantages, and substitute possibilities.
- ❖ **Improved Recipe Understanding:** Readers may better grasp recipe instructions and modify them to fit their preferences or dietary constraints by being aware of the terminologies and ingredients. This information ensures that dishes follow the DASH diet guidelines while also encouraging creativity in the kitchen.
- ❖ **Education on Healthy Choices:** By informing readers about the advantages of different components for their health, the glossary supports the cookbook's educational component. For instance, outlining the benefits of potassium-rich foods like bananas for controlling blood pressure or stressing the advantages of using olive oil rather than butter for heart health.
- ❖ **Developing Confidence:** In the end, the glossary helps readers become more confident in their capacity to follow the DASH diet. Readers may confidently plan meals, shop for groceries, and cook delectable, heart-healthy foods that complement their health objectives if they are familiar with nutritional words and ingredients.

The inclusion of a glossary in the cookbook guarantees that readers will get a greater comprehension of the DASH diet's guiding principles in addition to learning how to prepare wholesome meals. This instructional element improves the whole experience by enabling people to adopt a healthier lifestyle by making educated food choices.

Conclusion

Virgil famously said, "The greatest wealth is health," which sums up the main goals of the DASH diet. The 60-day meal plan is a major accomplishment that should be acknowledged and celebrated. It's essential to acknowledge your accomplishments if you want to stay motivated and keep the progress you've achieved. Here's how to maintain your focus on heart health while acknowledging and building on your accomplishments.

Acknowledging accomplishments is more than simply giving someone a pat on the back; it also entails reflecting on the trip, valuing the work put in, and recognizing the real advantages realized. This might be reduced blood pressure, weight reduction, heightened energy, or just feeling better all over. Take a minute to record your improvement. Put your original objectives, difficulties, and strategies for overcoming them in writing. To see the difference, compare your statistics from before and after. Talking about your achievements with loved ones may also make you feel accomplished and inspire others to help or even accompany you on your path.

Beyond the 60-day food plan, maintaining a heart-healthy lifestyle requires implementing important practices that promote long-term health. Maintaining consistency is essential. Maintain your daily implementation of the DASH diet by giving whole foods, lean proteins, low-fat dairy, and limiting salt consumption priority. Make meal preparation and planning a regular part of your schedule to guarantee that you have wholesome alternatives accessible at all times. This lessens the likelihood that, when you're pressed for time or energy, you'll turn to less healthful options.

Another crucial element of a heart-healthy lifestyle is physical exercise. Frequent exercise helps control weight, lower blood pressure, and enhance cardiovascular health in addition to the DASH diet. Aim for two or more days a week of muscle-strengthening exercises in addition to at least 150 minutes of moderate-intensity aerobic activity, such as brisk walking. To make exercising a sustainable and pleasurable part of your routine, choose something you like doing.

Despite being important for general health, staying hydrated is often neglected. Your heart is one of the systems in your body that is supported by water. Try to have eight 8-ounce glasses of water a day, or more depending on the weather and amount of activity you engage in. Making hydration more attractive may be achieved by limiting sugary drinks and choosing water, herbal teas, or infused water with fruits and herbs.

Maintaining your emphasis on mindful eating—which you probably started with the DASH diet—is important. This entails eating mindfully, relishing every meal, and paying attention to signals of hunger and fullness. Eating with awareness reduces the risk of overindulging and promotes a positive connection with food. It's also critical to practice self-compassion and flexibility. You may sometimes indulge in meals that don't follow the DASH recommendations, and that's OK. Moderation and balance are essential. Make the most of your meals nutritious and healthful, but don't feel bad about indulging in occasional pleasures.

Heart health is significantly maintained by practicing stress management. Both blood pressure and general well-being may be adversely affected by ongoing stress. Include stress-relieving practices in your everyday routine, such as yoga, meditation, deep breathing techniques, or even enjoyable and peaceful pastimes. Making sleep a priority is also essential. Try to get between seven and nine hours of good sleep every night to promote general health and well-being.

See your doctor regularly to track your progress and make any dietary or lifestyle changes that may be required. To keep informed about your heart health, monitor your blood pressure, cholesterol, and other pertinent health metrics.

Having a strong support network may help you continue to live a heart-healthy lifestyle. Be in the company of loved ones, friends, or others who support your health objectives. They may support you, provide wholesome cooking ideas, engage in physical activities with you, and assist in holding you responsible.

Gaining more knowledge about heart health and diet will enable you to make wise choices. Keep abreast with the most recent findings and suggestions, and for individualized advice, think about speaking with a dietitian or nutritionist.

To avoid boredom and to keep things interesting, vary up your meals. Try out new dishes, a variety of fruits and veggies, and different cooking techniques. This guarantees that you acquire a variety of nutrients and also makes eating more pleasurable.

Even while consuming nutritious meals, pay attention to portion proportions. Weight gain and other health problems might still result from overeating. To control portions, use gadgets like food scales or measuring cups, and pay attention to your body's signals of hunger and fullness.

An approach to eating that is balanced includes making plans for the odd splurge. Permit yourself to sometimes indulge in your favorite meals. This may lessen the chance of binge eating and help avoid feelings of deprivation.

Think back to the improvements you've seen since beginning the DASH diet. Better health indicators, more vitality, a happier mood, and an overall sense of well-being are all results of your diligence and hard work. Make good decisions going forward by drawing inspiration from these insights.

Lastly, think about how you may motivate others by sharing your DASH diet experience. Tell them about yourself, provide guidance and encouragement, and inspire them to make better decisions. Taking up the cause of heart health advocacy may help your community develop a more comprehensive wellness culture.

To sum up, acknowledging your accomplishments, keeping up the habits you've developed, and adopting a well-rounded and knowledgeable approach to eating and living are all important parts of celebrating your success on the DASH diet and leading a heart-healthy lifestyle. Although your path to heart health is not over, you are well-equipped to keep making decisions that promote your longevity and well-being because of the information, resources, and inspiration you have obtained. Your adherence to the DASH diet is evidence of your lifetime pursuit of improved health, and the advantages you have already seen are just the start.

Acknowledgments

Creating this book has been a deeply rewarding journey, and I owe a great deal of gratitude to many individuals whose support and contributions have been invaluable.

First and foremost, I would like to extend my heartfelt thanks to my family and friends for their unwavering encouragement and belief in me throughout this project. Your love and support have been my greatest source of strength.

A special thank you to my editor, whose keen eye for detail and insightful feedback helped shape this book into its final form. Your expertise and dedication to excellence have been truly inspiring.

I am immensely grateful to the team at Avalon Publishing House , who believed in this project from the very beginning. Your guidance and support have been instrumental in bringing this book to life.

To the numerous health and nutrition experts who generously shared their knowledge and expertise, thank you for your invaluable contributions. Your insights have enriched the content of this book and ensured that it is both accurate and practical.

I would also like to acknowledge the individuals and families who have adopted the DASH diet and shared their experiences with me. Your stories of transformation and success have been a tremendous source of inspiration and have reinforced the importance of this work.

A sincere thank you to my friends and colleagues who provided feedback on early drafts, offered words of encouragement, and celebrated each milestone along the way. Your support means the world to me.

Finally, to the readers of this book, thank you for embarking on this journey towards better health and wellness. I hope this book serves as a valuable resource and guide, and that it inspires you to achieve your health goals and live your best life.

With deep gratitude,

Kelley Hamilton

About the Author

Kelley Hamilton is a dedicated nutritionist and passionate advocate for heart-healthy living. With a background in nutritional science and years of experience helping individuals improve their health through diet and lifestyle changes, Kelley has become a trusted voice in the field of health and wellness. She holds a degree in Nutritional Science from University of Warwick and is a certified nutritionist, specializing in heart health and weight management.

Kelley's commitment to health and nutrition is driven by her personal journey and professional experiences. Having witnessed the transformative power of a balanced diet in her own life and the lives of her clients, she is dedicated to sharing the benefits of the DASH diet with a wider audience. Her approach is grounded in scientific research, and she is known for her ability to translate complex nutritional concepts into practical, actionable advice.

In addition to her work as a nutritionist, Kelley is a prolific writer and educator. She has authored numerous articles and guides on various aspects of nutrition, healthy eating, and lifestyle management. Her clear, engaging writing style and evidence-based recommendations have earned her a loyal following among readers seeking reliable health information.

When she's not working with clients or writing about nutrition, Kelley enjoys experimenting with new recipes, hiking, and spending time with her family. She believes that healthy eating should be enjoyable and accessible to everyone, and she is passionate about helping others achieve their health goals through delicious, nutritious food.

"The Science-Backed DASH Diet Meal Prep for Beginners" is Kelley's latest endeavor, combining her expertise in nutrition with her love for meal planning and cooking. Through this book, she aims to empower readers to take control of their health, lower their blood pressure, and enjoy a lifetime of heart-healthy eating.

Grocery LIST

Vegetables:

Fruits:

Meat and Poultry:

Seafood:

Dairy and Eggs:

Grains and Breads:

Canned Goods:

Snacks and Treats:

Condiments:

Miscellaneous Items:

Grocery LIST

| Vegetables: | Fruits: | Meat and Poultry: |

| Seafood: | Dairy and Eggs: | Grains and Breads: |

| Canned Goods: | Snacks and Treats: | Condiments: |

| Miscellaneous Items: |

__ / __ / ____

TRACK TODAY

	BEFORE	AFTER
BREAK FAST		
LUNCH		
SNACK		
DINNER		

NOTE

MOOD:

  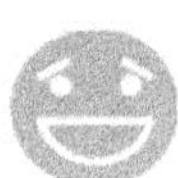   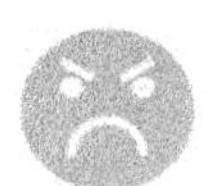

__ / __ / ____

TRACK TODAY

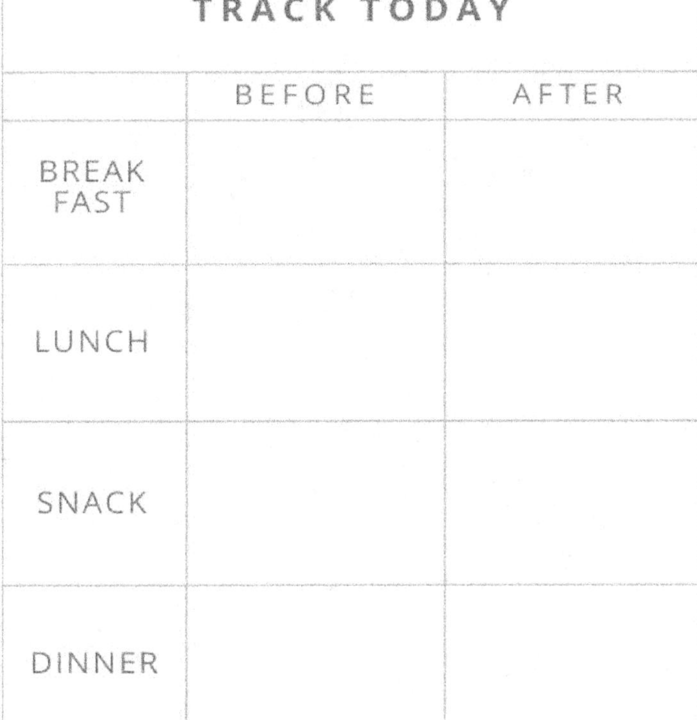

	BEFORE	AFTER
BREAK FAST		
LUNCH		
SNACK		
DINNER		

NOTE

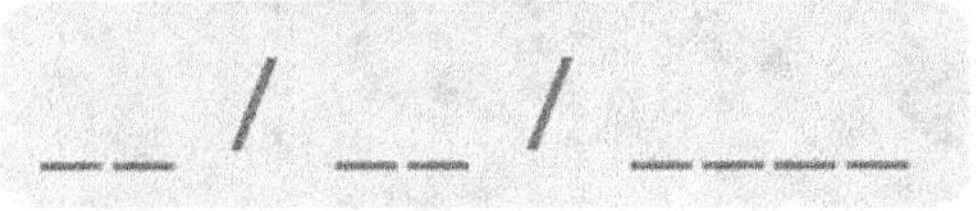

MOOD:

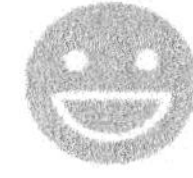 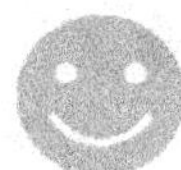 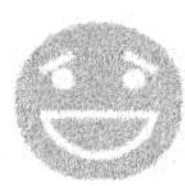  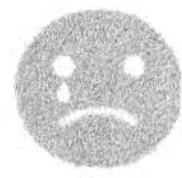 

__ / __ / ____

TRACK TODAY

	BEFORE	AFTER
BREAK FAST		
LUNCH		
SNACK		
DINNER		

NOTE:

MOOD:

 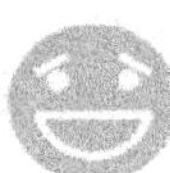   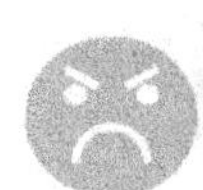

__ / __ / ____

TRACK TODAY

	BEFORE	AFTER
BREAK FAST		
LUNCH		
SNACK		
DINNER		

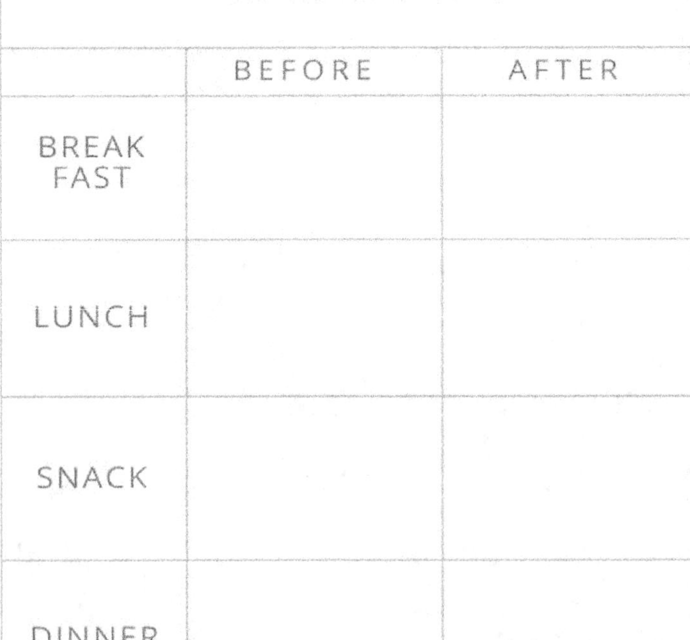

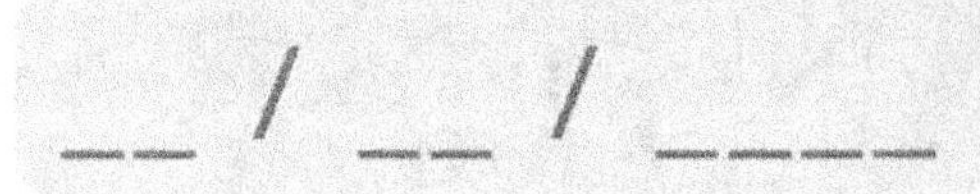

NOTE:

MOOD:

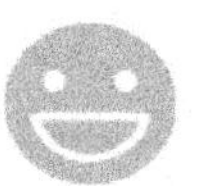 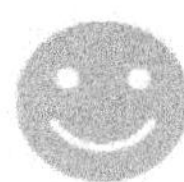 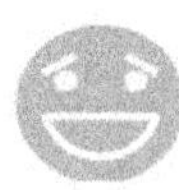   

FRIDAY

TRACK TODAY

	BEFORE	AFTER
BREAK FAST		
LUNCH		
SNACK		
DINNER		

NOTE:

MOOD:

 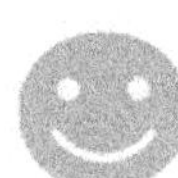 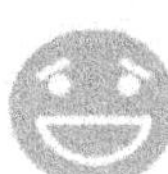   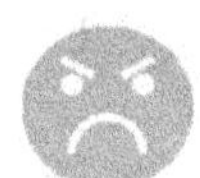

SATURDAY

TRACK TODAY

	BEFORE	AFTER
BREAK FAST		
LUNCH		
SNACK		
DINNER		

NOTE:

MOOD:

 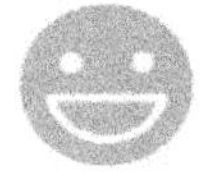 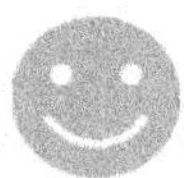 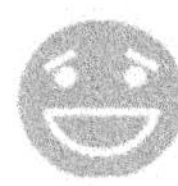  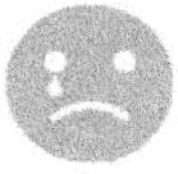 

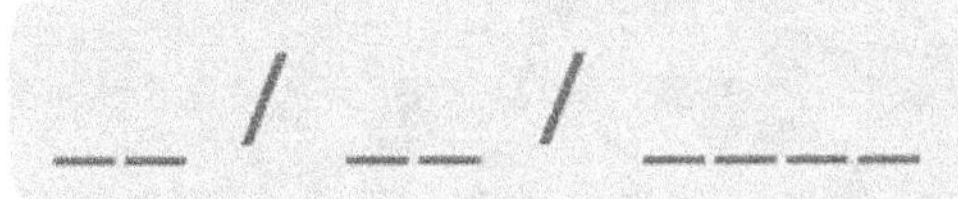

__ / __ / ____

TRACK TODAY

	BEFORE	AFTER
BREAK FAST		
LUNCH		
SNACK		
DINNER		

NOTE:

MOOD:

 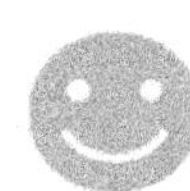 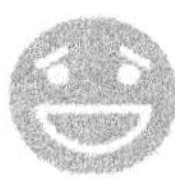  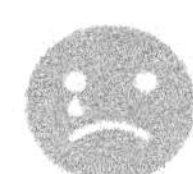 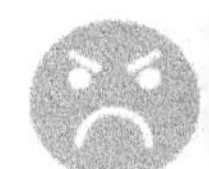

WEEKLY SUMMARY

Weight Tracker

START	END

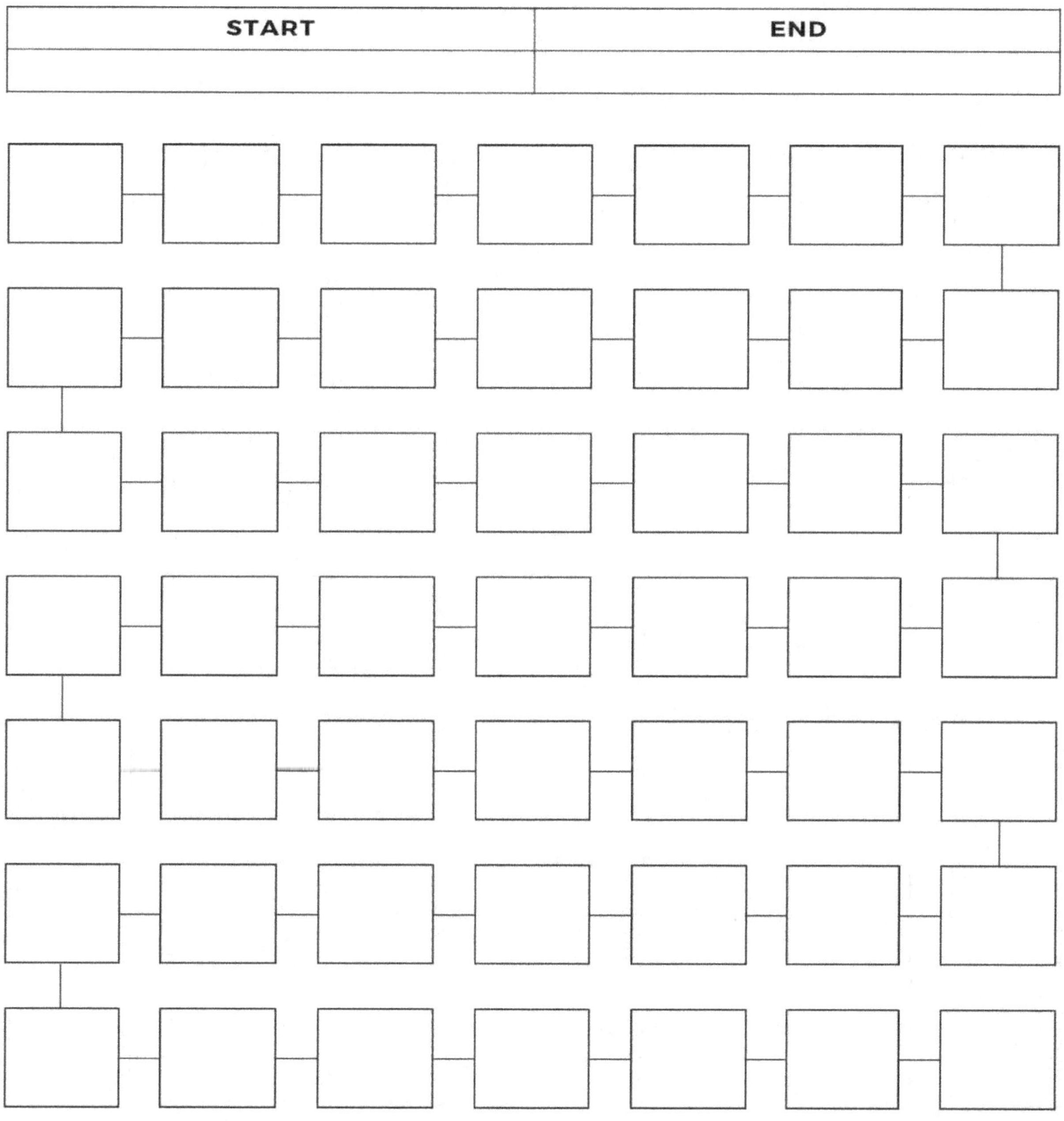

Weight Tracker

START	END

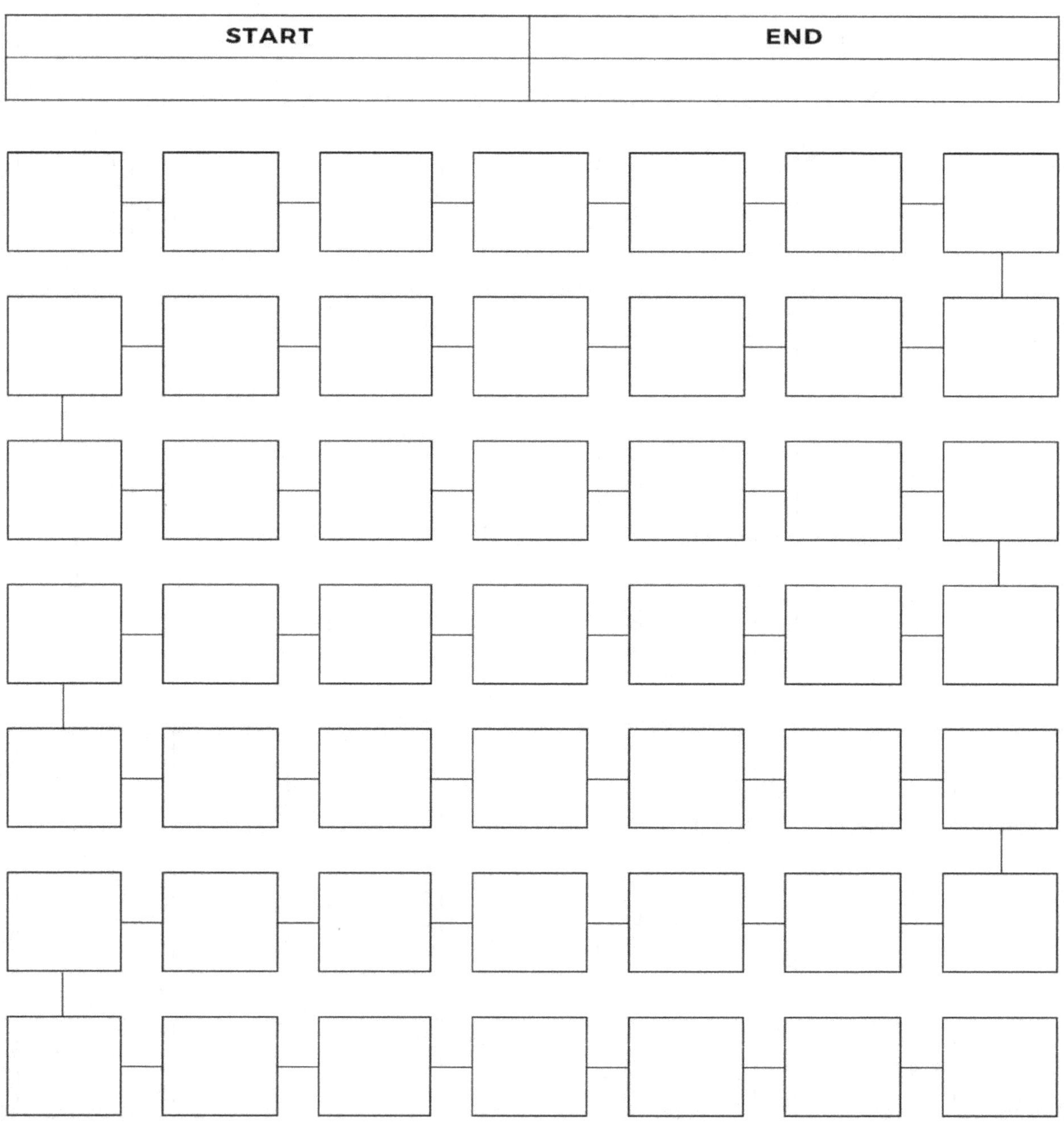

Weight Tracker

START	END

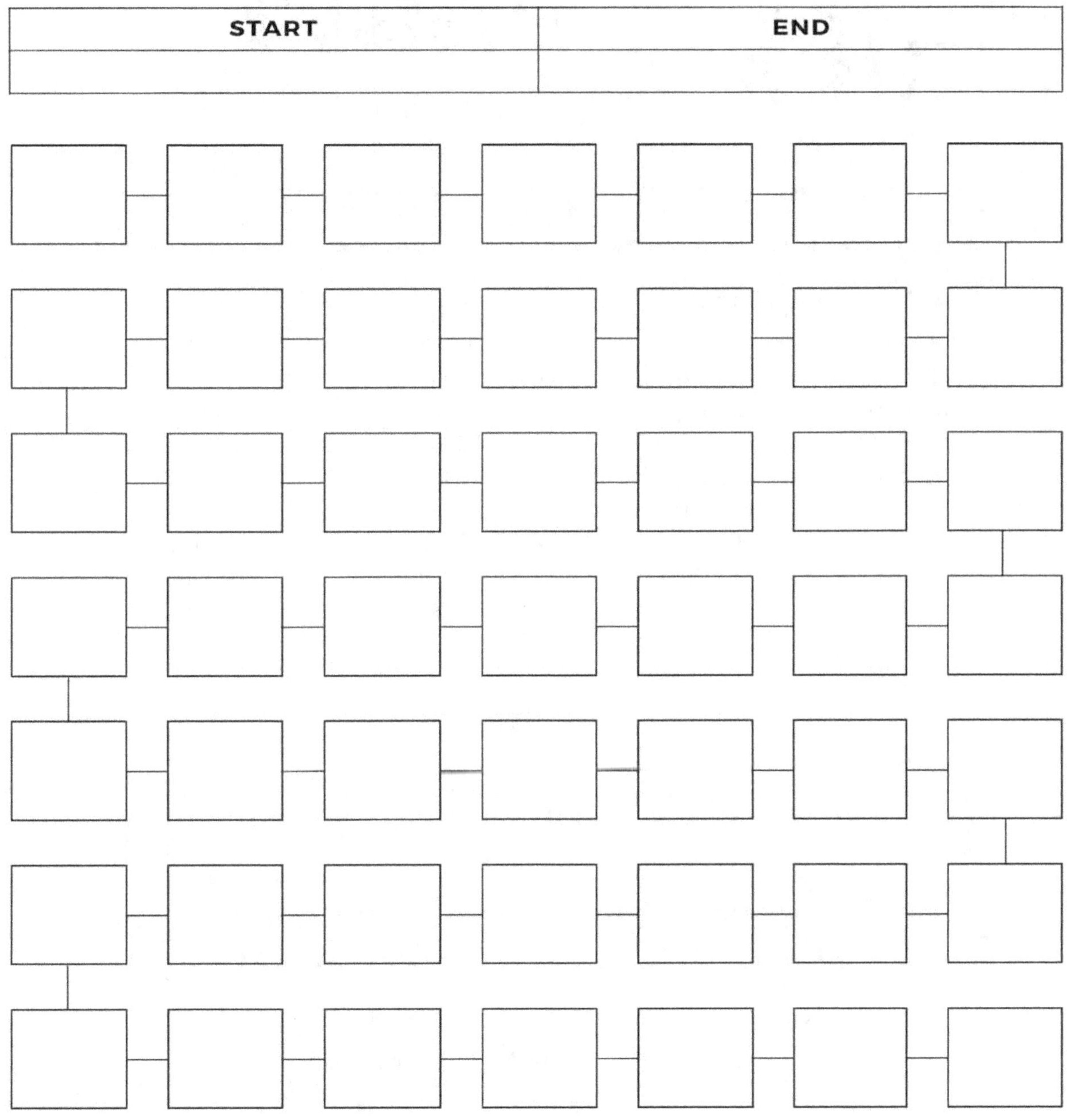

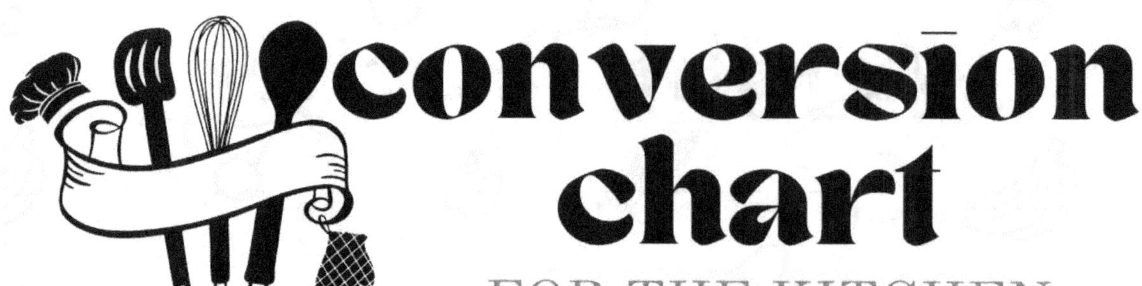

VOLUME MEASUREMENT CONVERSIONS

Cups	Tablespoons	Teaspoons	Milliliters
1/16 cup	1 tbsp	1 tsp	5ml
1/8 cup	2 tbsp	3 tsp	15 ml
1/4 cup	4 tbsp	6 tsp	30 ml
1/3 cup	5 1/3 tbsp	12 tsp	60 ml
1/2 cup	8 tbsp	16 tsp	80 ml
2/3 cup	10 2/3 tbsp	24 tsp	120 ml
3/4 cup	12 tbsp	32 tsp	160 ml
1 cup	16 tbsp	36 tsp	180 ml
		48 tsp	240 ml

1 QUART =
2 pints
4 cups
32 ounces
950 ml

1 PINT =
2 cups
16 ounces
480 ml

1 CUP =
16tbsp
8 ounces
240 ml

1/4 CUP =
4 tbsp
12 tsp
2 ounces
60 ml

1 TBSP =
3 tsp 1/2
ounce
15 ml

COOKING TEMPERATURE CONVERSIONS

Celcius/Centigrade	$F=(C \times 1.8) + 32$
Fahrenheit	$C=(F-32) \times 0.5556$

BAKING INGREDIENT CONVERSIONS

BUTTER

Cups	Grams
1/4 cup	57 grams
1/3 cup	76 grams
1/2 cup	113 grams
1 cup	227 grams

PACKED BROWN SUGAR

Cups	Grams	Ounces
1/4 cup	55 grams	1.9 oz
1/3 cup	73 grams	2.58 oz
1/2 cup	110 grams	3.88 oz
1 cup	220 grams	7.75 oz

ALL-PURPOSE FLOUR / CONFECTIONER'S SUGAR

Cups	Grams	Ounces
1/8 cup	16 grams	563 oz
1/4 cup	32 grams	1.13 oz
1/3 cup	43 grams	1.5 oz
1/2 cup	64 grams	2.25 oz
2/3 cup	85 grams	3 oz
3/4 cup	96 grams	3.38 oz
1 cup	128 grams	4.5 oz

GRANULATED SUGAR

Cups	Grams	Ounces
2 tbsp	25 grams	89 oz
1/4 cup	67 grams	1.78 oz
1/3 cup	50 grams	2.37 oz
1/2 cup	100 grams	3.55 oz
2/3 cup	134 grams	4.73 oz
3/4 cup	150 grams	5.3 oz
1 cup	201 grams	7.1 oz